Quality Management In Anatomic Pathology

Promoting Patient Safety Through Systems Improvement And Error Reduction

College of American Pathologists Surgical Pathology, Autopsy, Cytopathology, and Histotechnology committees

Raouf E. Nakhleh, MD
Patrick L. Fitzgibbons, MD
Editors

Caryn L. Tursky
CAP Staff Editor & Designer

Library of Congress Control Number: 2005924466
ISBN: 0-930304-86-1

Advancing Excellence

College of American Pathologists
325 Waukegan Road
Northfield, Illinois 60093
800-323-4040

Contributing authors

Richard W. Brown, MD

Memorial Hermann Healthcare System
Houston, Texas

David K. Carter, MD

St. Mary's/Duluth Clinic Health System
Duluth, Minnesota

Cheryl M. Coffin, MD

University of Utah
Primary Children's Medical Center
Salt Lake City, Utah

Diane D. Davey, MD

University of Kentucky Medical Center
Lexington, Kentucky

Marcella F. Fierro, MD

Virginia Department of Health
Office of Chief Medical Examiner
Richmond, Virginia

Patrick L. Fitzgibbons, MD

St. Jude Medical Center
Fullerton, California

Deborah Kay, MD

Virginia Department of Health
Office of Chief Medical Examiner
Richmond, Virginia

Virginia A. LiVolsi, MD

University of Pennsylvania Hospital
Philadelphia, Pennsylvania

Dina R. Mody, MD

The Methodist Hospital
Houston, Texas

Raouf E. Nakhleh, MD

Mayo Clinic College of Medicine
Jacksonville, Florida

Mary Ann Sens, MD, PhD

University of North Dakota School of Medicine
Grand Forks, North Dakota

John E. Tomaszewski, MD

University of Pennsylvania Hospital
Philadelphia, Pennsylvania

Theresa M. Voytek, MD

Hartford Hospital
Hartford, Connecticut

Mark A. Weiss, MD

TriHealth Laboratories
Good Samaritan Hospital
Cincinnati, Ohio

Acknowledgements

The editors and contributing authors wish to acknowledge the following current and past committee members, CAP staff, and others who also contributed to the chapters in this book.

Surgical Pathology

Oyedele Adewale Adeyi, MBBS
Lawrence J. Burgart, MD
David P. Frishberg, MD
Mary Beth Beasley, MD
Kumarasen Cooper, MBChB, PhD
Joel E. Haas, MD
Jerry W. Hussong, MD, DDS
Mary L. Nielsen, MD
Michael J. O'Brien, MD
Gary Pearl, MD
Douglas Murphy, CAP staff

Autopsy

Kevin E. Bove, MD
John J. Buchino, MD
Edward C. Klatt, MD
David L. Gang, MD
John Sinard, MD, PhD
Stephen A. Geller, MD
Richard Michael Conran, MD, PhD, JD
Kim Collins, MD
Jeremy S. Ditelberg, MD
William Ahrens, MD
Elizabeth Burton, MD
Keri Gonzalez, CAP staff

Cell Markers

Kumarasen Cooper, MBChB, PhD
Richard N. Eisen, MD
Andrew L. Folpe, MD
Eric D. Hsi, MD
Michael D. Linden, MD
Rodney T. Miller, MD
Robert R. Rickert, MD
Raymond R. Tubbs, DO
Douglas Murphy, CAP staff

Cytopathology

George G. Birdsong, MD
Terence J. Colgan, MD
William Frable, MD
Ann T. Moriarty, MD
Marianne U. Prey, MD
Andrew Renshaw, MD
Mary R. Schwartz, MD
Janet Stastny, DO
Emily E. Volk MD
Lisa Fatheree, CAP staff
Jennifer Haja, CAP staff

Histotechnology

Freida L. Carson, PhD, HT(ASCP)
Janice LeMond, HT, HTL(ASCP)
Lena T. Spencer, MA, HT(ASCP), HTL, QIHC
Marilyn Gamble, HTL(ASCP)
Sue E. Lewis, BS, HTL(ASCP)
Vinnie Della Speranza, MS, HTL(ASCP)
Jill Kachin, CAP staff
Jacques Mobille, CAP staff

Contents

Chapter 4   Strategies for error reduction and prevention in surgical pathology   33

Chapter 5   Defining and handling errors in surgical pathology   41

Chapter 6   Quality improvement plan components and monitors   45

Chapter 7   Quality management in the histology laboratory   77

Introduction

Raouf E. Nakhleh, MD

Quality Management in Anatomic Pathology: Promoting Patient Safety Through Systems Improvement and Error Reduction has been produced by the College of American Pathologists (CAP) to provide pathologists with a framework for a complete and organized approach to quality improvement in the anatomic pathology laboratory. This new text is based on the CAP's *Quality Improvement Manual in Anatomic Pathology,* which was originally published in 1988 and has served as a valuable resource for pathologists throughout the world.

Since the last *QI Manual* was published in 2002, there has been increased public pressure to continuously assure patient safety and reduce medical errors. This text provides more detailed analyses of error reduction strategies in anatomic pathology and includes guidelines and quality assurance and improvement monitors for areas not previously discussed, including immuno-histochemical and molecular pathology laboratories. There is also a more extensive discussion of issues related to histology laboratories.

Quality Management in Anatomic Pathology maintains the structure and organization of the previous manuals. Our goals are to review error reduction strategies that have been well established in other industries, discuss how some of these strategies may be applied to the anatomic laboratory, and provide valuable benchmark data that can be incorporated into routine quality monitors.

In keeping with the earlier CAP publications, this text provides pathologists with the tools necessary to develop and maintain a comprehensive quality improvement plan for anatomic pathology. Since the scope of pathology practice varies widely, the manual includes many different types of recommendations, not all of which are necessary for each laboratory. Although an attempt was made to be as complete as possible, new approaches or modifications of existing approaches to quality improvement continue to be tested and implemented. Consequently, not every discussion presented here is necessary for every lab, and no single plan should be considered comprehensive or definitive for all labs.

Historical perspective

The clinical laboratory, with its focus on accuracy and precision of analytic procedures, developed and implemented effective quality control measures earlier than anatomic pathology. Anatomic pathology as a specialty developed in the patient care setting, with an emphasis on clinical correlation, interpretation, and differential diagnosis. These activities lagged in traditional quality control testing. Quality assurance was brought into focus in this country during the 1980s when American manufacturers realized the quality gap between their products and those of Japanese producers. Prior to this, quality assurance was primarily the domain of industries with the potential for major disasters (eg, aviation). By many measures, the health care industry as a whole has only recently begun to adopt concepts of quality improvement and deal effectively with medical error. This is highlighted in the Institute of Medicine report on medical error,[1] which has stimulated greater focus on quality improvement, error reduction, and patient safety.

Traditionally, the analysis of quality has been divided into three levels: quality control, quality assurance, and quality improvement.

Quality control activities evaluate the uniformity of specific processes and basic functions to assure that they are operating within acceptable parameters. These processes include the ways in which laboratories accession, process, interpret, report, and retain submitted specimens. Quality control monitors are typically designed to compare the actual performance of the process with the process set forth in the departmental procedure manual. Examples of quality control activities in the anatomic pathology laboratory include such things as:

- Routine checking of instruments
- Maintaining temperature logs of water baths and cryostats
- Controls for special stains
- Maintaining procedures for obtaining specimens
- Determining the quality of sectioning and staining

Quality assurance, a term used to indicate a system designed with internal quality checks, encompasses a higher level of oversight and relies upon the collection of outcome data. Typically, these outcomes encompass multiple processes or procedures. These activities often monitor such things as report timeliness or diagnostic error rates. Examples of quality assurance monitors in anatomic pathology include:

- Frozen section accuracy
- Frozen section turnaround time
- Rate of specimen identification errors
- Diagnostic accuracy
- Completeness of information for tumor staging (eg, tumor size, status of surgical margins) included in the report.

Quality improvement activities seek to improve outcomes such as those listed above. Thus, a department's quality improvement goals might include such things as *reducing* diagnostic error rates, *shortening* turnaround time, and *improving* customer satisfaction. Quality improvement activities use quality assurance monitors to determine the effectiveness of an intervention. Typical steps in this process include:

1. Identify an indicator or process to improve.
2. Measure current level of performance for that process.
3. Determine target or desirable level of performance for that process.
4. Design and implement an intervention.
5. Re-evaluate level of performance for that process.
6. Repeat steps, as necessary, to achieve desired level of performance.

Focus on patient care

Pathology is not considered a primary care specialty, but is directly involved in patient care by helping to provide information that is essential for evaluation and management. Since many pathologists interact with patients infrequently, it can be easy to forget that the primary purpose of developing a quality improvement plan is to improve patient care. Regardless of the size or scope of a pathology practice, the primary goal of these activities must be to improve patient care.

The systems approach to quality improvement

The basis of a systems approach lies in accepting that most errors occur due to poor system design and not the individual working within that system. Mistakes are unintended human actions, and the natural response is to blame the individual for his or her action or inaction. Many of these errors are thought to be due to "latent system errors." Latent system errors are inadequacies of a system that are not manifested when a system is designed, but which ultimately result in errors or mistakes. Examples of latent system errors include inadequate staffing for a particular task or job, defective equipment, ineffective communication, and poor training. Many systems operate reasonably well until stresses are placed on the system. Those stresses may come in the form of more work than anticipated, unexpected absences, or unfamiliar situations, and increase the chance that employees, in their diligence to keep up with the work, will make mistakes.

While human fallibility can be mitigated with knowledge and training, most experts agree that this approach must be accompanied by system enhancements and modifications. Furthermore, focusing on individuals through blame and shame for having made mistakes is frequently counterproductive and can damage morale and trust, factors necessary for team-building and an effective workplace. Education and training in all areas, including error reduction strategies, must be conducted in a healthy nonpunitive environment. Effective error reduction must encompass critical analysis of the systems involved, with system redesign and enhancements encompassing proven techniques, as discussed in chapter 4.

While the essence of anatomic pathology remains tissue diagnosis, enhancements in obtaining, processing, and examining tissues, and in formatting and delivery of diagnostic reports have improved the overall quality of pathology practice. Pathologists should embrace system enhancements that reduce errors, increase efficiency, reduce costs, improve accuracy, and improve timeliness and completeness. The introduction and acceptance of synoptic reports is one example of a successful system enhancement that can improve patient care by reducing the chance of error. The evolution of information technologies has begun to transform many aspects of pathology and will likely drive further changes in our field. Pathologists should continuously strive to adopt such enhancements when they improve patient care.

Developing a quality program

Quality improvement activities consume a significant amount of laboratory resources. Developing and implementing an annual quality improvement plan requires coordinating the desired goals with the resources needed to carry it out. Since resources are often limited, quality improvement activities for any given year must be selected prudently. Just as a plan that is too limited to identify significant problems would be inadequate, attempting to accomplish too much can also result in incomplete or inadequate information.

Too often, quality assurance programs are thought of as isolated activities assigned to select individuals. In this view, quality assurance is often considered only as the quality assurance meeting is approaching and selected data have to be collected and presented. Ideally, quality assurance and improvement are incorporated into the overall mission of the department and are everyone's responsibility. Every individual in the department should be convinced that maintaining quality at each step leads to the best possible outcome.

In this manual, we have attempted to cover the areas traditionally considered quality improvement activities, namely, ongoing checks or monitors of systems and processes. However, one must remember that many individual elements are necessary for a quality program in anatomic pathology. A quality program requires competent and informed people at each level, continuous education, uniform methodology, uniform criteria and application of criteria where interpretation is necessary, orderly work flow, accommodating systems that assure tasks are easily and fully completed, ongoing checks or monitors of systems, regulatory compliance, and, finally, a product that meets the needs of customers. As such, quality assurance needs to be integrated into the normal daily workflow of the laboratory and should be considered part of everyone's job. Along with other responsibilities, written job descriptions should include a description of specific quality assurance responsibilities, and completion of these activities should be part of employment evaluations. This integration provides greater efficiency and makes quality improvement an integral part of the laboratory.

Reference

1. Kohn LT, Corrigan JM, Donaldson MS, eds. *To Err Is Human: Building a Safer Health System.* Washington DC: National Academy Press; 2000.

Designing a quality improvement plan

Raouf E. Nakhleh, MD

The plan

The College of American Pathologists (CAP) Laboratory Accreditation Program (LAP) requires laboratories to have a written quality improvement plan (LAP checklist item ANP.10000). This plan is most effective when it is simple and speaks to its mission in a direct way. Ideally, a document entitled, *"Quality Improvement Plan for Year _____,"* should be created annually (see Figure 2-1). This document should include an outline of the areas to be addressed and specific monitors to be performed. Each monitor should include benchmark levels with references from the literature or other sources to compare with your data. An institution should have a goal of improving on its own benchmarks as well as external benchmarks.

A mission statement

A quality improvement plan should have a defined mission that reflects departmental and institutional objectives. The mission statement, or quality assurance committee charge statement, could be the same as the department's mission statement (eg, "The Department will enhance patient care with timely, accurate, and complete surgical pathology diagnoses and reports"). Ideally, this statement should embody the values of the department and institution.

The test cycle (preanalytic, analytic, and postanalytic)

All diagnostic and analytic laboratories have a defined test cycle composed of preanalytic, analytic and postanalytic segments. Understanding this test cycle in anatomic pathology assists in identifying and isolating problems so that they can be more effectively addressed. Dividing pathology processes into test cycle components also provides an opportunity to organize the quality improvement plan into more manageable components.

Since problems can occur at every step of the test cycle, quality improvement plans must incorporate monitors to evaluate procedures in each segment. One must also realize that a monitor of processes in one segment may detect problems arising in one of the other two segments. For example, in monitoring reports for report completeness (postanalytic), one may find specimen identification errors (preanalytic). Recognizing the part of the test cycle in which the problem is occurring (eg, accessioning, not transcription) can lead to more effective solutions.

Priorities

The departmental quality improvement plan should strive to examine all aspects of the test cycle, but realizing the limitations of available resources, one must prioritize and put into place a multi-year plan. Pathologists must determine how many monitors can be effectively carried out in a given time frame and, accordingly, determine what can and should be done each year. Areas with the most frequent problems, or areas in which problems have the potential for being the most significant, are generally targeted before areas of lesser importance. Unfortunately, if resources or attention are not given to problem areas, accurate measurement will not occur, and it is likely that effective solutions will not be found. It is imperative that proper resources be devoted for each monitor or activity selected for that year's quality improvement plan.

Individual responsibility and timetable

For a plan to work, specific individuals should be responsible for specific tasks. In addition to clear deadlines, these individuals must be given adequate time to carry out these tasks. Insufficient time devoted to quality improvement activities will result in incomplete or misleading information and a poor plan. The timetable should include regular meetings of the appropriate institutional committee, which may be monthly, bimonthly, or quarterly. Specific monitors should be reported at each meeting. An annual planning meeting to assess the activities of the previous year and to determine which monitors should be carried forward and which should be stopped in favor of other monitors should also be considered.

Institutional concerns

The departmental quality improvement plan should reflect the needs of the institution that it serves. In devising an annual plan, a department must reflect on problems identified within the institution or where the laboratory may provide a solution. Clearly, problems perceived or known to arise from within the Pathology Department should be addressed, but one may also look to participate in quality improvement activities outside the laboratory, which provides an opportunity to be viewed as team players and problem solvers.

In creating a quality improvement plan, designate a monitor or monitors to be reported to the institutional quality committee. These monitors should have value in demonstrating the pathologists' attention to improving processes as well as departmental proficiencies and contributions to the institution. Examples may include frozen section correlation, turnaround time in a specific area, and physician satisfaction surveys.

External and internal benchmarks

The appropriate use of data is crucial to any quality improvement program. As data is collected, it ideally should be compared with internal or external benchmarks and trended over time. These comparisons will determine whether a problem exists and whether a monitor needs to be continued. There are many sources for this type of data. In chapter 6, we have attempted to include references to such sources. In an ideal setting, improvement should be continuous and therefore a moving target.

Figure 2-1. Example of an anatomic pathology quality improvement plan

Quality Improvement Plan for Year 2005

A. Mission statement.

"The Quality Improvement Program in Anatomic Pathology of ANYWHERE HOSPITAL covers surgical pathology, cytopathology, and autopsy pathology. To help achieve the hospital's vision, we strive continually to improve patient and physician satisfaction, reduce the cost of care, improve outcomes, and reduce delays in every aspect of care. This plan is intended to measure, assess, and improve the quality of service we provide, in order to fulfill our mission of providing the best possible care for our patients."

B. Quality Improvement Committee. Membership and meeting schedule.

Dr. ____, chair of the Quality Improvement Committee of the Department of Pathology, is responsible for the preparation of reports and quality monitors.

The Quality Improvement Committee (Drs. X_____, Y_____, and Z_____; and Laboratory supervisors A_____, B_____, and C_____) will assist in the preparation and review of these reports and quality monitors. The Committee meets on the second Friday of each month at noon in the Pathology library and issues monthly/quarterly reports to the Hospital Quality Council and Medical Executive Committee.

Once a year, the Quality Improvement Committee meets to review the prior year's quality improvement program and to structure the program for the following year.

C. Specific monitors for the current year (2005).

Details of each of these monitors, including methods of data gathering, frequency of analysis, and benchmarks, are described in the departmental policy and procedure manuals.

Monitors	Individual Responsible	Reporting Schedule	Benchmark Level Used	Reference for Benchmark Data
Preanalytic				
Specimen identification				
Unsatisfactory cytology specimens by physician				
Analytic				
Diagnostic accuracy				
Correlation of frozen section diagnosis with final diagnoses				
Cytologic-histologic correlation				
Postanalytic				
Report completeness				
Check of electronic report delivery				
Turnaround Time				
Biopsy specimens TAT				
Autopsy final report TAT				
Customer Satisfaction				
Overall AP survey				

Documentation of action taken to correct any deficiencies detected by the quality improvement program is maintained along with the monthly reports and monitors. Follow-up review is carried out to ensure that deficiencies, once detected, are corrected. Results of the follow-up review are maintained with those of the original studies.

Figure 2-1. Example of an anatomic pathology quality improvement plan (continued)

Quality Improvement Plan for Year 2005

D. Data reported to Institutional QI Committee.

Monitors	Reporting Schedule	Benchmark Level Used	Reference for Benchmark Data
Specimen identification			
Correlation of frozen section diagnosis with final diagnoses			
Autopsy final report TAT			
Overall AP satisfaction survey			

Regulatory compliance

David K. Carter, MD

Introduction

The Clinical Laboratory Improvement Amendments of 1988 (CLIA '88) mandate periodic surveys of clinical laboratories in the United States to ensure compliance with regulatory standards, to promote reliable diagnostic services, and to provide laboratory reimbursement eligibility from federal and state funding programs. The Centers for Medicare and Medicaid Services (CMS), an agency of the US Department of Health and Human Services, surveys laboratories for compliance. CMS also gives approved status to other organizations to conduct surveys. Laboratories that are accredited by approved organizations are deemed by CMS to meet the requirements of CLIA '88 and do not have to undergo a separate inspection by CMS. Approved organizations include but are not limited to the College of American Pathologists (CAP) through its Laboratory Accreditation Program (LAP). Under CLIA '88, clinical laboratory tests are classified as waived, minimally complex, or highly complex. Anatomic pathology services are included in the highly complex test category, which requires stringent quality control and quality assurance policies and procedures.

Other federal regulations also affect anatomic pathology practice. The Safe Medical Devices Act of 1990 requires device-user facilities to report to the manufacturer instances where a medical device has apparently caused or contributed to a patient's death, serious illness, or serious injury. Devices subject to tracking under this regulation are listed in the *Federal Register*[1] and reprinted in Exhibit 3-1 (see CAP LAP checklist items GEN.20370, 20371). Pathologists who examine medical devices should document serial numbers, if present.

Standards produced by the Occupational Safety and Health Administration (OSHA) of the US Department of Labor cover potential occupational exposure to pathogens and hazardous chemicals. OSHA instructs employers to strive to provide a workplace free of recognized hazards, and to provide employees appropriate warnings of hazards and access to personal protective equipment. Details should be included in the department's policy manual, and compliance is addressed in the CAP LAP checklists (Tables 3-1 and 3-2). Acceptable formaldehyde levels should be documented, and periodic monitoring may be indicated in some situations. Medical waste disposal and newer environmental regulations of reagents such as mercury should also be addressed (GEN.70512). Radioactive material processing and disposal (eg, sentinel lymph node and associated tissues, specimens with brachytherapy seeds) should follow policies established with the institutional radiation safety officer (ANP.11275). Anatomic pathology labs should also note slide and block disposal guidelines and periodic cleaning and disinfection of cryostats (ANP.24250).

The US Centers for Disease Control and Prevention (CDC) and state health departments also provide reporting guidelines and issue periodic alerts to laboratories, to assist in recognition of potential bioterrorism agents or emerging pathogens (eg, severe acute respiratory syndrome [SARS]).[2] Such activities serve a critical public health service and should be addressed in laboratory policies.

The Health Insurance Portability and Accountability Act of 1996 (HIPAA) mandates new regulations to govern privacy, security, and electronic transactions for identifiable health care information.[3] These regulations became effective April 2003. For anatomic pathology laboratories, this primarily affects the postanalytic phases of practice. Some aspects of HIPAA are not directly applicable to pathologists or laboratories because of their "indirect treatment relationship" with the patient (ie, delivering diagnostic reports to another provider rather than directly to the patient). However, consent issues and de-identification of materials for education and research must be addressed in laboratory policies. The CAP provides on-line references regarding HIPAA issues facing laboratories.[4] Pathologists should work closely with their organizations' legal counsel, privacy officer, and information technology specialists to ensure HIPAA compliance.

With advances in molecular diagnostics, issues of genetic testing and associated regulations should also be addressed. Anatomic pathology specimens may be utilized for identification of specific gene or chromosomal abnormalities. These abnormalities may be isolated (acquired) somatic mutations but may also be related to germline defects and thereby point to heritable risk factors for neoplasia, such as hereditary nonpolyposis colorectal cancer syndrome or *BRCA* tumor suppressor gene mutations in breast-ovarian cancer syndromes. Results of such testing may carry ramifications for family members in addition to patients. Some states require documentation of genetic counseling prior to specific genetic testing. Although regulations continue to evolve,[5,6] laboratories may wish to consider additional consent forms prior to genetic testing and/or close cooperation with clinical providers for such documentation.

The Food and Drug Administration (FDA) has issued regulations for immunohistochemical studies using analyte specific reagents (ASRs)[7,8] (see Exhibit 3-2). Since late 1998, laboratories must include a disclaimer on reports when ASRs have been active ingredients of tests developed in house. Reagents are specified as Class I, II, or III, depending on whether they are used adjunctively with conventional histopathologic examination or whether independently reportable diagnostic information is generated, as with HER2/*neu*. This is addressed in the CAP LAP checklist (ANP.12425), and recommended disclaimer language is included in the ASR section in Exhibit 3-2. In addition to ASRs, the CAP is currently updating reporting guidelines applicable to immunohistochemical reagents when used as predictive markers or to determine eligibility for newer targeted therapies made from specific antibodies (proposed ANP.22200-22900).

The Joint Commission on Accreditation of Healthcare Organizations (JCAHO), in addition to its survey activities, monitors sentinel events,[9] defined as unexpected occurrences involving death or serious physical or psychological injury, or risk thereof. Reportable sentinel events relevant to the anatomic pathology laboratory include:

- Unanticipated death or the major permanent loss of function, not related to the natural course of the patient's illness or underlying condition
- Surgery on the wrong patient or wrong body part

When these occur, a focused audit and root cause analysis of both laboratory and system-wide procedures must be completed. Some institutions may also mandate root cause analysis for "near-miss" occurrences, defined as adverse outcomes that fall short of sentinel events. Appropriate procedures should be in place for prompt reporting of sentinel and near-miss events identified in the anatomic pathology laboratory.

The JCAHO survey mechanisms as of January 1, 2004, include new Tracer Methodology, wherein selected patients' care is tracked through the multiple hospital departments involved in diagnosis and treatment. This appropriately focuses on overall systems processes rather than specific incidents. Accordingly, pathology groups should review how their individual policies interface with nursing, medical records, surgery, and other departments' operational procedures.

In addition to laboratory oversight through CLIA, OSHA, HIPAA, the FDA, and the JCAHO, individual states may have specific laboratory regulations. These regulations may have ramifications for licensure, consultation practices, and the use of telepathology. Specific guidelines, or requirements for privileges or credentialing, may also exist through policies set by local health care organizations and risk management committees. Some third-party payers also may have requirements in test ordering and reporting practices, which groups may need to address to ensure reimbursement for pathology services. Other accrediting agencies, such as the American College of Surgeons Commission on Cancer, have guidelines for pathology reporting of new malignancies, which also affect laboratory practice.

Benchmarks to assess a department's quality initiatives can be obtained through the CAP Q-Probes program. Other mechanisms, such as trend analysis and intradepartmental peer comparisons of observed versus expected diagnostic rates, may be utilized.[10] Specifics are addressed elsewhere in this manual, particularly in chapter 6.

JCAHO medical staff standards for hospitals state that "at the time of renewal of privileges, the organized medical staff evaluates individuals for their continued ability to provide quality care, treatment, and services for the privileges requested as defined in the medical staff bylaws." Therefore, pathologists may be required to submit competency documentation of their practice to institutional credentialing/staff appointment committees. Quality assurance data on individual performance may be a component of this documentation but must be used in the context of peer group comparisons. This is best done when using multiple performance parameters including but not limited to turnaround times, diagnostic concurrence or discordance rates, and customer satisfaction or customer complaints.

In summary, for accreditation purposes and to ensure regulatory compliance, anatomic pathology policies must carefully outline standard operating procedures and strive for consistency in the complex and variable aspects of preanalytic, analytic, and postanalytic phases of diagnostic services. Approaches to achieve this are discussed below. Summary tables of the CAP LAP checklists follow, including LAP question number references, to serve as a guide for the main topics detailed later in this manual.

Preanalytic phase compliance

Guidelines for specimen submission
(GEN.40000-40125, 40700, 40750)

In general, all tissues, fluid specimens, cytologic preparations, and other specimens obtained from patients are submitted to the pathology laboratory for examination. This allows both identification of suspected or unsuspected diseases and independent documentation of procedures and specimen types. Guidelines for specimen submission must be made available to operating rooms, endoscopy suites, clinics, nursing units, and off-site physicians' offices. The specific details of these guidelines will vary with each institution and may include information about fixation, times of service for specimens requiring special handling, and clinical information to be included with the specimen. Groups also may wish to consider specimen-specific order forms or guidelines for particular biopsies (eg, liver, breast, nerve, kidney) for correlation with necessary clinical data and/or imaging findings.

Exempted and gross-only specimens
(ANP.10016, 10032, 11550, 12200)

Some specimens may not require gross and/or microscopic examinations, and institutions may decide to exempt certain specimens from submission to the pathology laboratory or from a requirement for routine microscopic examination. Specific exemptions from pathologic evaluation, if any, must be determined jointly by members of the medical staff and the pathologist(s), documented in institutional policy, and reviewed for compliance with state and federal regulations, including the Safe Medical Devices Act of 1990 (see Exhibit 3-1). A 1997 CAP Q-Probes study assessed policies and exempted specimen practices in 413 institutions.[11] The CAP Surgical Pathology Committee has also published guidelines for specimens exempted from pathologic examination (see Exhibit 3-3).[12]

Specimens exempted from submission to the pathology laboratory must still be documented in the medical record, which is usually the responsibility of the attending physician who performed the procedure. Also, the relevant department should maintain a log of tissues and medical devices not submitted for pathologic evaluation, with information about final disposition (eg, returned to physician or patient, archived in risk management department, discarded).

Specimens exempted from routine microscopic evaluation should also be documented in institutional policy. Lists of such specimens (eg, "gross-only" list) should be developed jointly by pathologists and other members of the medical staff.[11] Gross-only examination has been challenged on occasion by third-party payers as representing a documentation or quality assurance practice rather than a pathologic examination (ie, medical service). Hence, the pathology report should clearly document the relevant findings, such as the absence of features that would require microscopic examination. When unusual findings are encountered during gross examination, the pathologist must exercise professional discretion to perform histologic examination or other studies, as indicated.

Specimen labeling and rejection
(GEN.40750)

Specimen submission guidelines should include requirements for specimen labeling and requisition form completion. Since most anatomic pathology specimens are unique and irreplaceable, rejection criteria must be considered carefully. A serious effort to resolve ambiguous identification should be applied before specimens are rejected. Increased attention to labeling of specimen laterality (right versus left) should also be encouraged. This may already be a requirement in many medical centers as an additional safety check regarding prevention of "wrong site" surgeries.

Requisition form retention
(ANP.12500)

Pathology requisition forms must be retained for at least 2 weeks and can serve as critical documentation should any question arise as to the accuracy of the information transcribed. Options include retaining the original requisitions, either with file copies of patient reports or in a separate file, or scanning the forms into an electronic archive.

Analytic phase compliance

Gross examination personnel
(ANP.11600-11640, 11670)

Pathologists should determine with technical personnel and pathologists' assistants the specimen types that may be grossly described, dissected, and sampled by nonpathologists. Educational requirements and a mechanism for continued competency assessment are important considerations. With growing use of telepathology services in centers possibly not routinely staffed on site by pathologists, such competency is of even greater importance to ensure standard of care.

Tissue distribution

The pathologist plays a key role in tissue distribution and specimen triage, while ensuring that adequate material for diagnosis is retained. Providing tissue for special procedures or research protocols should be at the discretion of the pathologist responsible for the case, should not compromise patient care, and should be performed according to institutional policies, including institutional review board (IRB) requirements. To the extent possible, cases requiring special handling are best scheduled when necessary resources are available. Patient consent and patient or family privacy issues regarding materials used for research or education purposes and genetic testing considerations are discussed above (HIPAA compliance).

Specimen integrity during processing
(ANP.21050, 21100, 21150, 21200)

The laboratory should particularly consider mechanisms to decrease potential specimen or tissue block-slide labeling mix-ups during processing. Relatively simple procedures, such as not accessioning like specimens in consecutive numbers and providing accurate descriptions of number and size of tissue fragments placed in cassettes, are worthwhile. Color coding of specimens with inks or cassette-slide labels may also be employed. Prelabeling of slides or blocks may be an acceptable practice provided that procedures are in place for appropriate use. The increased application of automated methods and bar coding technology should assist in ensuring specimen integrity through the analytic phase of pathology services. (See also chapter 4.)

Intradepartmental and extradepartmental consultations
(ANP.10150, 10200, 10250, 30050)

Procedures for obtaining and documenting intradepartmental and extradepartmental consultations should be described in the departmental policy manual. The CAP Surgical Pathology Committee has been made aware of the diverse methods by which groups may document such activities. Careful consideration of true *consultations* versus quality assurance *reviews* is a useful endeavor, as documentation of such either in or out of patient record or as internal departmental records only should be a policy-driven and consistent process. Extradepartmental consultations are usually identified based on pathologist-perceived diagnostic difficulty or lack of consensus opinion following intradepartmental consultation. Although not usually generated because of diagnostic difficulty, extradepartmental consultations also occur when patients take their slides to another institution for a second opinion. While these can serve as a useful quality measure, departments may wish to distinguish this form of consultation from the former. Departments may institute other mechanisms for generating outside consultation of selected cases.

A policy requiring, or at a minimum strongly suggesting, review of outside pathology materials prior to surgery or other therapeutic intervention is encouraged. Consistency in procedures for internally generated pathology consultations on such outside material is also encouraged (ie, formal written report versus informal and often poorly documented "curbside" slide reviews for clinicians). Slides and blocks should be promptly returned to the originating pathologist in most cases, or a request for permission to retain such materials should be issued.

Copies of pathology reports generated on outside material should always be sent to the original pathology department. In the event of significant disagreement, the case should be promptly discussed with the referring pathologist.[13,14] Pathology departments have discretion in whether the results of such unsolicited second reviews should be routinely incorporated into a formal report. However, in situations of significant diagnostic discrepancies following such reviews, a supplemental report to reconcile such differences is encouraged. Many groups track such reviews as an effective quality assurance monitor.

Correlation of ancillary studies, including immunohistochemistry, with pathologic findings (ANP.12400, 12425, 54000)

Results of immunohistochemical stains, in situ hybridization studies, and other ancillary studies, should be clearly documented in the pathology report. For immunohistochemistry, tissue fixation, antibody, and in some instances (eg, HER2/*neu*, estrogen and progesterone receptor assays) antibody clone number should be specified. Other ancillary studies, such as molecular diagnostic tests, flow cytometry, and electron microscopy, may be handled similarly. Ancillary test results that are received after the final report has been issued should be reported in a supplemental report. This addendum should also correlate the findings with the original morphologic impression and reconcile any discrepancies. Studies once considered "ancillary" now often provide the most accurate diagnosis or may provide a more specific tumor subtype (eg, World Health Organization [WHO] leukemia and lymphoma classifications). Original reports based on morphology should be worded in such a manner as to later allow final definitive diagnosis as an addendum or supplemental report, without potential discordant results (see also "Pathology reporting," under "Postanalytic phase compliance"). Mechanisms to facilitate correlation of bone marrow smears and histologic sections, particularly if prepared and examined in separate areas of the laboratory or medical center, should also be developed (proposed modifications to ANP.12400 and HEM.36250).

Many reagents formerly used only as ancillary diagnostic tools now serve as prognostic markers or components of free-standing tests that directly influence use of targeted cancer therapies (eg, CD117, HER2, HER1, CD20). Choice of such reagents may invoke necessary ASR disclaimer statements. Particular cancer treatment trial regulations or accreditation by outside organizations may also mandate tighter regulations or extra-level proof of competency through participation in appropriate surveys and/or more stringent statistics tracking, such as trends analyses of the laboratory's results. The CAP is also currently updating reporting and procedural guidelines for immunohistochemistry when reagents are utilized as predictive markers or targeted-therapy determinants (proposed ANP.22200-22900).

Intraoperative consultation and frozen sections
(ANP.10100, 11800-12075, 24250)

Frozen section policies are often a key monitor for a department's quality assurance plan (see chapter 6). Additional considerations in this area include limiting infectious risk through cryostat decontamination and guidelines for handling of potentially infectious unfixed specimens.[15] Cryostat decontamination has recently been elevated to a Phase II requirement (ANP.24250).

Policies describing when frozen section examinations will be performed can be developed in conjunction with surgery and other clinical departments. For example, frozen sections of very small breast lesions or potentially infectious tissues may not yield helpful information, may compromise further pathologic evaluation, or may pose a risk to patients or personnel. Exceptions occur, so flexibility and patient care needs are important considerations.

A policy regarding permanent slide preparations from the frozen tissue remnant should be in place. Many departments do this routinely, or have exceptions based on specimen type (eg, en face margin sections, wherein the most representative material is present in original frozen section [ANP.12075]).

Postanalytic phase compliance

Pathology reporting
(ANP.10100-10200, 12000-12425; GEN.43500, 43700-43730)

Pathology departments routinely issue several different types of pathology reports, which should be defined in the departmental procedure manual to improve communication and promote better understanding among pathologists and other medical staff members.

A **final** pathology report is a completed report that becomes part of the permanent medical record and includes the final diagnosis and all necessary diagnostic information. Pathology reports are issued for cases in which only a gross examination is performed ("gross-only") or, more commonly, when both gross and microscopic examinations are performed.

A **provisional** (or preliminary) report is used when the pathologist anticipates a delay in producing the final report. This may occur for a number of reasons, such as the need to obtain special stains or other ancillary studies, review of archival or outside material, or the decision to obtain expert consultation. A provisional report should describe what is pending before the final report can be issued and should clearly indicate that the findings are preliminary and may be changed in the final report.

An **addendum** report is issued when new information becomes available after the final report has been submitted. Newly obtained clinical information, findings on additional histologic sections or review of archival material, the results of special studies such as immunohistochemistry or molecular diagnostics, and the results of consultations may be included in an addendum report. An addendum report may or may not change the original diagnosis. When issued following a provisional report, the addendum report may actually represent the final report.

A **revised** (or amended) report is issued when the final diagnosis changes or other important pathologic information becomes available. The reasons for the revision must be explained in the report and the clinician(s) notified, because a revised report may significantly affect patient care.

Some departments also define a **corrected** report, which is issued when transcription, patient identification, specimen site, or other related reporting errors occur. A corrected report differs from a revised report because the diagnosis remains unchanged. Corrected reports should be clearly identified and the reasons for the correction included in the report. The clinician(s) should be notified when corrections are likely to influence patient care.

As anatomic pathology reports generally contain textual data (versus most clinical lab results), it may be unnecessary to repeat the entire original report in the revised report. However, it is imperative that the originally reported information be included in some fashion in the revision.

Some laboratories use the term "addendum report" to refer to any pathology report issued subsequent to the final report. Regardless of the specific terms used, communication with the treating physicians and clear explanation of the purpose of the new report are essential. Assessing revised report frequency can be a useful monitor, but revised or amended report rates alone are inadequate measures of diagnostic error.[16]

An alert or urgent-diagnosis call policy should also be established based on specimen types or unusual diagnoses (ANP.12175). Although not usually within the strict definition of a "critical value" (ie, imminently life threatening [GEN.41320]), certain surgical pathology findings may warrant pathologists' or their designees' increased efforts to reasonably ensure clinicians' receipt of such results.

Electronic-only reporting of pathology results is becoming more common in the realm of integrated electronic medical record systems. Pathologists should work closely with their health information service departments to ensure integrity of pathology reports when released in electronic fashion. Formats and readability of reports through various modalities should be audited periodically (see chapter 6). Some method of electronic verification of clinician receipt should also be sought, although it is recognized that this is a shared responsibility with our clinical colleagues to close the loop and ensure pathology reports have been read. HIPAA regulations also note increased scrutiny of facsimile (faxed) reports' format and cover-sheet privacy statements.

Slide/tissue retention and send-out
(ANP.11550, 12500, 23700)

The institution has a responsibility to store patient materials safely for a reasonable amount of time. The CAP requires minimum retention times for slides, blocks, and reports, as listed in the LAP checklist (ANP.12500) (Table 3-3). The older practice of carefully sealing paraffin blocks prior to storage is overly burdensome and not necessary in most instances. Policies regarding loan of tissue blocks or slides to outside institutions, such as centralized pathology review centers for clinical trials or tumor banks, are required. If blocks are sent out, laboratories should consider retaining some diagnostic materials, such as original or representative slides. In general, blocks and slides should be returned to the original institution when outside studies are completed. This should be done promptly so as to not disrupt patient care (ANP.10250) (see Exhibit 3-4, "Stewardship of pathologic specimens"). If special studies are performed on outside tissue blocks, slides may either be retained at the referral center or returned to the original institution. This decision may need to be made on a case-by-case basis; in general, diagnostic materials should remain close to the center of current patient care.

Duration of slide retention in the LAP checklist refers to conventional (permanent) stains. Fluorescence stains do not retain diagnostic changes due to loss of fluorescence or other factors. The retention time for such slides should be determined by local policy. Alternative documentation, such as digital photography, may be considered but is not currently mandated. Similarly, individual departments should determine decisions regarding retention of photos or digital images of pathology materials.

Departments or medical centers may also require documentation of patient consent prior to release of materials. Consent likely is not needed if for legitimate continuance of care issues, but may be required in some situations (refer to HIPAA regulations and institutional privacy officer).

Release of tissue specimens to patients should take into consideration potential chemical and biological hazards. Such policies should be developed in cooperation with a hospital's legal counsel and risk management department, and should take into account an institution's operative or admission permits' language and applicable state guidelines regarding patient ownership of specimens. Tissues or other materials for release should be appropriately packaged and labeled, including biohazard tags. Chemical and biologic hazards remain at a low but finite level even in fixed and washed specimens,[17] and many institutions have adopted a "no release" policy on tissue, with exceptions for religious, cultural, and forensic considerations. Use of a specimen release form is encouraged to document patients' receipt, understanding, and acceptance of exposure risks. Gross photographs may be offered in lieu of specimen release.

Tissue disposal
(ANP.11275, 12500, 23700, 24200, 24300, 27150, 33500, 34000-34150, 42100, 57070; GEN.70600-70700, 73000, 73100)

Disposal of wet tissues, paraffin blocks, and glass slides should follow policy, including established time intervals, as specified in the CAP LAP checklist. Specifics of disposal (ie, laboratory sink, general waste water system, incineration, or other mechanisms for biohazard material disposal) should follow institutional, local, and state regulations. In the current era of sentinel lymph node biopsies, disposal of radioactive material (both the sentinel node and the resected tumor tissue) should be coordinated with the institution's radiation safety officer.[18] A procedure for Creutzfeldt-Jakob disease should be in place; the CAP LAP checklist references provide useful guidelines (ANP.24300, 34150). Mercury disposal issues have been noted earlier in this chapter.

Questions about retention of certain materials, such as silicone breast prostheses, are commonly received by CAP staff. The CAP Surgical Pathology Committee developed recommendations for handling prosthetic breast implants in 1994. It is suggested that patients be informed that explanted devices will be stored for a specified period of time and then discarded, unless requested otherwise by the patient. This notification may be accomplished though the operative consent form, among other mechanisms. A reasonable time period for retention would range from a minimum of 30 days to a maximum of 6 to 12 months. Indefinite retention is not warranted in most cases.[19]

Reports and records retention
(ANP.12500, 33500; GEN.20372, 30200)

Reports should be retained for at least 10 years. Regarding quality assurance documents, separate requirements for surgical pathology are not specified, but a useful guideline is 2 years, similar to quality control documents retention in general laboratory and cytology departments. As discussed above, if quality assurance documents are not maintained indefinitely, it is important that they be clearly specified as quality assurance documents and not internal consultation records, as the latter should be retained as mandated for original pathology reports. There is no requirement for keeping working drafts, raw data checklists, or other preliminary materials other than requisition forms.

Miscellaneous regulatory items
(GEN.13806 – 20373)

Above items from the general laboratory checklist are particularly relevant to anatomic pathology. All policies and procedures in pathology, as in other areas of the laboratory, should be subject to a formal document management or control system, ensuring that written policies and procedures are current, relevant documents have been reviewed by appropriate personnel, discontinued policies/procedures are retained for 2 years, etc (GEN.20372). Customer satisfaction surveys (physicians or patients, as appropriate) should be performed. The overall quality management plan should be reviewed and modified, as appropriate, based on key areas such as large volume tests, particularly critical patient care procedures, and areas which have had past problems or are prone to quality issues based on published studies or institutional history. The pathology quality management program should also be coordinated with other hospital services' quality initiatives (GEN.15354). Policies and signage regarding laboratory employee reporting of quality concerns are also required (GEN.20365, 20366)

Summary

Tables 3-1 and 3-2 have been adapted from the CAP LAP checklists (ANP September 2004, GEN December 2004 editions) and are intended to facilitate integration of a laboratory's quality efforts with CAP LAP accreditation requirements. The LAP checklist questions and references are available in electronic form via www.cap.org. These are an invaluable resource to laboratories and provide an efficient reference to quality laboratory practice parameters. Some laboratories have further integrated electronic policy manuals by utilizing computer network hyperlinks and cross-references from an intranet-based checklist item directly to the appropriate procedure in an electronic policy manual.[20]

The following tables include the checklist numbers and applicable phases of diagnostic testing (preanalytic, analytic, postanalytic), followed by a statement of each question's content and indexed chapters for further details on the subject contained in this manual. The items are arranged first by analytic process order (Table 3-1) and then by numerical order (Table 3-2).

Table 3-1. Checklist regulatory items arranged by phase in the test cycle

Phase	Checklist Number	Brief Description	Chapter/Page
From Anatomic Pathology (ANP) Checklist			
Preanalytic	10016, 10032	Specimen examination list: exempt and gross-only	3/12
Preanalytic, Analytic	21050, 21100, 21150, 21200	Identification of specimen maintained through processing; blocks, slides, and slide labels identified and legible	3/13
Analytic	08216	Formaldehyde safety	3/9
Analytic	10050	Review of previous material with current case	—
Analytic	10100	Frozen section reconciled in final report	6/50
Analytic	10150, 10200	Intra- and extradepartmental consults documented	3/13
Analytic	11275	Radioactive specimens	3/9
Analytic	11500	Specimen identification maintained	3/13
Analytic	11600 – 11640	Gross examination personnel	3/13
Analytic	11800, 11850	Frozen section processing, turnaround time, and reporting	6/50,66
Analytic	12150	Routine case turnaround time 48 hours	6/68
Analytic	12250	Key to tissue blocks' designation in report	—
Analytic	12350	Information for grading/staging neoplasms in report	6/61
Analytic	12400	Correlation of special studies with general findings and reconciliation in final report	3/14
Analytic	12425	Immunohistochemistry: ASR, IVD, RUO, etc	3/10,25
Analytic	22250 – 22950	Immunostaining procedures and quality control	8/93-108
Analytic	22956 – 22986	FISH, ISH procedures	—
Analytic	24200 – 24300, 27150	Infectious material handling and disposal; CJD precautions; slide/block disposal	3/17
Analytic, Postanalytic	07328	Slides/blocks for consultation or legal proceedings	3/16,28
Analytic, Postanalytic	12000, 12050, 12075	Frozen section reported in final, frozen section slides retained, and permanent slide made of residual frozen material	3/15
Postanalytic	02000	Peer educational program enrollment	—
Postanalytic	10000	Quality management (QM) program defined	2/5-7
Postanalytic	10250	Review of outside material, report copy to original pathologist	3/13
Postanalytic	11550	Retention of wet tissue 2 weeks after report	3/17,23
Postanalytic	12175	Unexpected findings: timely communication	3/16

Table 3-1. Checklist regulatory items arranged by phase in the test cycle (continued)

Phase	Checklist Number	Brief Description	Chapter/Page
Postanalytic	12500	Records retention times for tissue, slides, blocks, reports	3/16,23
Postanalytic	22950	Retention of immunostained slides	3/16,23
Postanalytic	23750	Retention of blocks	3/16,23
Autopsy Items			
Preanalytic	31070, 31100	Consent, coroner jurisdiction	—
Analytic	30050	Autopsy intra- and extradepartmental consultations documented	10/156
Analytic	33100 – 33150	Autopsy turnaround time (provisional report in 48 hours; final report in 60 days)	10/154
Analytic	34000, 34150	Autopsy infectious precautions; CJD precautions	—
Analytic	42100	Autopsy safety compliance	—
Analytic	57070	EM reagents disposal	—
Postanalytic	30000	QM program for autopsy	10/153-182
Postanalytic	30100	Autopsy results used to correlate with clinical	10/156,176
Postanalytic	30150	Autopsy results used in overall institution QM plan	10/156,159,179
Postanalytic	33500	Retention of autopsy records and materials	3/17,23
Postanalytic	30575	Unexpected findings reported	—
From General (GEN) Checklist			
Preanalytic	40000 – 40125, 40350, 40400	Instructions for specimen collection	3/11
Preanalytic	40512, 40522	Infectious materials packaging and shipping	3/11
Preanalytic, Analytic	40550, 40600, 40700, 40750 – 40940	Details of specimen identification and tracking during receipt and testing procedures	3/12
Preanalytic, Postanalytic	41350, 41370, 41400, 41440	Mechanisms for choosing and reporting results from reference labs	—
Analytic	41470	Turnaround time for testing (service levels) defined	6/65-69
Analytic	44650	Computer downtime procedures	—
Analytic	70000 – 73100	Safety, includes: radioactive, formalin, liquid nitrogen, personal protective devices, latex, mercury, others	3/9
Postanalytic	10000	External audit, proficiency testing used	—
Postanalytic	13806 – 20369	Quality management issues	—
Postanalytic	15354	QM coordination with other hospital services	2/6
Postanalytic	20316	Quality key indicators monitored	6/45-71

Table 3-1. Checklist regulatory items arranged by phase in the test cycle (continued)

Phase	Checklist Number	Brief Description	Chapter/Page
Postanalytic	20370 – 20380	FDA-required device-related adverse events reporting, document control system in place	3/24
Postanalytic	30200	QC records retention 2 years	3/12,17
Postanalytic	40950 – 41330	Details of reporting format, parameters, ordering physician, urgent result notification mechanisms	3/15
Postanalytic	41480	Retention of laboratory records and materials	3/17
Postanalytic	43500	Verify format of printed reports	3/17, 6/61-63
Postanalytic	43650, 43730,	Corrected reports clearly specified as such, original report retained 2 years, sequential corrections documented	3/17
Postanalytic	50800	Monitoring quality of laboratory results, including reference laboratory results	2/5-7, 6/45-71

Table 3-2. Checklist regulatory items arranged by numerical order

Checklist Number	Phase	Brief Description	Chapter/Page
From Anatomic Pathology (ANP) Checklist			
02000	Postanalytic	Peer educational program enrollment	—
07328	Analytic, Postanalytic	Slides/blocks for consultation or legal proceedings	3/16,28
08216	Analytic	Formaldehyde safety	3/9
10000	Postanalytic	Quality management (QM) program defined	2/5-7
10016, 10032	Preanalytic	Specimen examination list: exempt and gross-only	3/12
10050	Analytic	Review of previous material with current case	—
10100	Analytic	Frozen section reconciled in final report	6/50
10150, 10200	Analytic	Intra- and extradepartmental consults documented	3/13
10250	Postanalytic	Review of outside material, report copy to original pathologist	3/13
11275	Analytic	Radioactive specimens	3/9
11500	Analytic	Specimen identification maintained	3/13
11550	Postanalytic	Retention of wet tissue 2 weeks after report	3/17,23
11600 – 11640	Analytic	Gross examination personnel	3/13
11820 – 11850	Analytic	Frozen section processing, turnaround time, and reporting	6/50,66

Table 3-2. Checklist regulatory items arranged by numerical order (continued)

Checklist Number	Phase	Brief Description	Chapter/Page
12000, 12050, 12075	Analytic, Postanalytic	Frozen section reported in final, frozen section slides retained, and permanent slide made of residual frozen material	3/15
12150	Analytic	Routine case turnaround time 48 hours	6/68
12175	Postanalytic	Unexpected findings: timely communication	3/16
12250	Analytic	Key to tissue blocks' designation in report	—
12350	Analytic	Information for grading/staging neoplasms in report	6/61
12400	Analytic	Correlation of special studies with general findings and reconciliation in final report	3/14
12425	Analytic	Immunohistochemistry: ASR, IVD, RUO, etc	3/10,25
12500	Postanalytic	Records retention times for tissue, slides, blocks, reports	3/16,23
21050, 21100, 21150, 21200	Preanalytic, Analytic	Identification of specimen maintained through processing; blocks, slides, and slide labels identified and legible	3/13
22250 – 22950	Analytic	Immunostaining procedures and quality control	8/93-108
22950	Postanalytic	Immunostained slides retention	3/16,23
22956 – 22986	Analytic	FISH, ISH procedures	—
23750	Postanalytic	Retention of blocks	3/16,23
24200 – 24300, 27150	Analytic	Infectious material handling and disposal; CJD precautions; slide/block disposal	3/17

Autopsy Items

Checklist Number	Phase	Brief Description	Chapter/Page
30000	Postanalytic	QM plan for autopsy	10/153-182
30050	Analytic	Autopsy intra- and extradepartmental consults documented	10/156
30100	Postanalytic	Autopsy results used to correlate with clinical	10/156,176
30150	Postanalytic	Autopsy results used in overall institution QI Plan	10/156,159,179
30575	Postanalytic	Unexpected findings reported	—
31070, 31100	Preanalytic	Consent, coroner jurisdiction	—
33100 – 33150	Analytic	Autopsy turnaround time (provisional report in 48 hours; final report in 60 days)	10/154
33500	Postanalytic	Retention of autopsy records and materials	3/17,23
34000, 34150	Analytic	Autopsy infectious precautions; CJD precautions	—
42100	Analytic	Autopsy safety compliance	—
57070	Analytic	EM reagents disposal	—

Table 3-2. Checklist regulatory items arranged by numerical order (continued)

Checklist Number	Phase	Brief Description	Chapter/Page
From General (GEN) Checklist			
10000	Postanalytic	External audit, proficiency testing used	—
13806 – 20369	Postanalytic	Quality management issues	—
15354	Postanalytic	QM coordination with other hospital services	2/6
20316	Postanalytic	Quality key indicators monitored	6/45-71
20370 – 20380	Postanalytic	FDA-required device-related adverse events reporting, document control system in place	3/24
30200	Postanalytic	QC records retention 2 years	3/12,17
40000 – 40125, 40350, 40400	Preanalytic	Instructions for specimen collection	3/11
40512, 40522	Preanalytic	Infectious materials packaging and shipping	3/11
40550, 40600, 40700, 40750 – 40940	Preanalytic, Analytic	Details of specimen identification and tracking during receipt and testing procedures	3/12
40950 – 41330	Postanalytic	Details of reporting format, parameters, ordering physician, urgent result notification mechanisms	3/15
41350, 41370, 41400, 41440	Preanalytic, Postanalytic	Mechanisms for choosing and reporting results from reference labs	—
41470	Analytic	Turnaround time for testing (service levels) defined	6/65-69
41480	Postanalytic	Retention of laboratory records and materials	3/17
43500	Postanalytic	Verify format of printed reports	3/17, 6/61-63
43650, 43730	Postanalytic	Corrected reports clearly specified as such, original report retained 2 years, sequential corrections documented	3/17
44650	Analytic	Computer downtime procedures	—
50800	Postanalytic	Monitoring quality of lab results, including reference lab results	2/5-7, 6/45-71
70000 – 73100	Analytic	Safety, includes: radioactive, formalin, liquid nitrogen, personal protective devices, latex, mercury, others	3/9

Table 3-3. Minimum requirements for surgical pathology retention* (ANP.12500)

Accession log records	2 years
Wet tissue (stock bottle)	2 weeks after final report
Paraffin blocks	10 years
Glass slides and reports	10 years

* Providing these are not less stringent than state and federal regulations

Exhibit 3-1. Safe Medical Devices Act of 1990

Complete list of devices required for tracking under the Safe Medical Devices Act of 1990[1]

1. Permanently implantable devices:

   - Vascular graft prostheses

   - Vascular bypass (assist) devices

   - Implantable pacemaker pulse generator

   - Cardiovascular permanent pacemaker electrode

   - Annuloplasty ring

   - Replacement heart valve

   - Automatic implantable cardioverter/defibrillator

   - Tracheal prosthesis

   - Implanted cerebellar stimulator

   - Implanted diaphragmatic/phrenic nerve stimulator

   - Implantable infusion devices

2. Life-sustaining or life-supporting devices:

   - Breathing frequency monitors (apnea monitors)

   - Continuous ventilator

   - CD-defibrillator and paddles

3. FDA-designated devices:

   - Silicone inflatable breast prosthesis

   - Silicone gel-filled breast prosthesis

   - Silicone gel-filled testicular prosthesis

   - Silicone gel-filled chin prosthesis

   - Silicone gel-filled angel chik reflux valve

   - Electromechanical infusion pumps

Exhibit 3-2. Analyte specific reagents (ANP.12425)

Analyte specific reagents (ASRs) are antibodies, both polyclonal and monoclonal, specific receptor proteins, ligands, nucleic acid sequences, and similar reagents which, through specific binding or chemical reaction with substances in a specimen, are intended for use in a diagnostic application for identification and quantification of an individual chemical substance or ligand in biological specimens.

By definition, an ASR is the active ingredient of an in-house-developed ("home brew") test system. ASRs may be obtained from outside vendors or synthesized in-house. ASRs from outside vendors are supplied individually. They are not bundled with other materials in kit form, and the accompanying product literature does not include any claims with respect to use or performance of the reagent. Class I ASRs in use in the anatomic pathology laboratory include some antibodies for immunohistochemistry and nucleic acid probes for FISH and ISH.

Class I ASRs are not subject to preclearance by the US Food and Drug Administration or to special controls by FDA. Thus, if the laboratory performs patient testing using Class I ASRs obtained or purchased from an outside vendor, federal regulations require that the following disclaimer accompany the test result on the patient report: "This test was developed and its performance characteristics determined by (laboratory name). It has not been cleared or approved by the US Food and Drug Administration."

The CAP recommends additional language such as, "The FDA has determined that such clearance or approval is not necessary. This test is used for clinical purposes. It should not be regarded as investigational or for research. This laboratory is certified under the Clinical Laboratory Improvement Amendments of 1988 (CLIA '88) as qualified to perform high complexity clinical laboratory testing."

The above disclaimer is not required when using reagents that are sold in kit form with other materials and/or an instrument, and/or with instructions for use, and/or when labeled by the manufacturer as Class I for in vitro diagnostic use (IVD), Class II IVD, or Class III IVD. Most antibodies used in immunohistochemistry are labeled "for in vitro diagnostic use" and thus do not require the disclaimer.

Antibodies, nucleic acid sequences, etc, labeled "Research Use Only" (RUO) purchased from commercial sources may be used in home brew tests only if the laboratory has made a reasonable effort to search for IVD or ASR class reagents. The results of that failed search should be documented by the laboratory director. The laboratory must establish or verify the performance characteristics of tests using Class I ASRs and RUOs in accordance with the Method Performance Specifications section of the Laboratory General checklist. The laboratory may put an ASR disclaimer on the pathology report for all immunostains, FISH and ISH studies collectively used in a particular case. Separately tracking each reagent used for a case and selectively applying the disclaimer to only the class I ASRs is unnecessary.

Exhibit 3-3. Surgical specimens to be submitted to pathology for examination

College of American Pathologists policy

Policy synopsis

Each institution, in conjunction with the pathologist and appropriate medical staff departments, should develop a written policy that addresses which specimens do not need to be submitted to the pathology department and which specimens may be exempt from a requirement for microscopic examination. The policy should clearly state that all specimens not specifically exempted must be submitted to the pathology department for examination. It should also state that a microscopic examination will be performed whenever there is a request by the attending physician, or when the pathologist determines a microscopic examination is indicated by the gross findings or clinical history. Each institution should have an alternative procedure for documenting the removal and disposition of any specimens or devices not submitted to pathology for examination. Recommendations about which specimens should routinely be submitted to pathology are included in the policy.

Policy

The College of American Pathologists has developed the following recommendations to help in determining what specimens should routinely be submitted to the pathology department for examination. These are intended only as suggestions and are not mandatory or a requirement for CAP accreditation.

Each institution, in conjunction with the pathologist and appropriate medical staff departments, should develop a written policy that addresses which specimens do not need to be submitted to the pathology department and which specimens may be exempt from a requirement for microscopic examination. This policy must be individualized for each institution and should take into account the diagnostic needs of the medical staff, the likelihood of significant findings in otherwise unremarkable specimens given the clinical situation, the reliability of procedures to ensure proper handling of specimens in surgery, and potential medicolegal implications. According to JCAHO Standards and CAP guidelines, this policy must be jointly determined by the pathologist and the institution's clinical staff.

The policy should clearly state that all specimens not specifically exempted must be submitted to the pathology department for examination. It should also state that a microscopic examination will be performed whenever there is a request by the attending physician, or when the pathologist determines a microscopic examination is indicated by the gross findings or clinical history. A pathology report should be generated for every specimen submitted to the pathology department for examination.

Creating two lists may be useful. One list should designate those specimens (if any) that are exempt from routine submission to the pathology department. A second list should specify those specimens that are to be submitted to pathology for gross examination but which are exempt from mandatory microscopic examination, ie, gross only examination.

The following are specimens that an institution may choose to exclude from routine or mandatory submission to the pathology department. There should be an alternative procedure for documenting the removal and disposition of any specimens or devices not submitted to pathology for examination. This is particularly important for any failed medical devices that may have contributed to patient injury, any failed device for which litigation is pending or likely, and for devices subject to tracking under the Safe Medical Devices Act of 1990 (see Exhibit 3-1).

- Bone donated to the bone bank
- Bone segments removed as part of corrective or reconstructive orthopedic procedures (eg, rotator cuff repair, synostosis repair, spinal fusion)
- Cataracts removed by phacoemulsification
- Dental appliances
- Fat removed by liposuction
- Foreign bodies such as bullets or other medicolegal evidence given directly to law enforcement personnel
- Foreskin from circumcisions of newborns
- Intrauterine contraceptive devices without attached soft tissue
- Medical devices such as catheters, gastrostomy tubes, myringotomy tubes, stents, and sutures that have not contributed to patient illness, injury or death
- Middle ear ossicles
- Orthopedic hardware and other radio-opaque mechanical devices provided there is an alternative policy for documentation of their surgical removal
- Placentas that do not meet institutionally specified criteria for examination[21]
- Rib segments or other tissues removed only for purposes of gaining surgical access, provided the patient does not have a history of malignancy
- Saphenous vein segments harvested for coronary artery bypass
- Skin or other normal tissue removed during a cosmetic or reconstructive procedure (eg, blepharoplasty, cleft palate repair, abdominoplasty, rhytidectomy, syndactyly repair), provided it is not contiguous with a lesion and the patient does not have a history of malignancy
- Teeth when there is no attached soft tissue
- Therapeutic radioactive sources
- Normal toenails and fingernails that are incidentally removed

It is recommended that the following specimens should be submitted to the pathology department for examination. These specimens often require only a gross examination. However, exceptions are at the pathologist's discretion.

- Accessory digits
- Bunions and hammertoes
- Extraocular muscle from corrective surgical procedures (eg, strabismus repair)
- Inguinal hernia sacs in adults*
- Nasal bone and cartilage from rhinoplasty or septoplasty
- Prosthetic breast implants[22]
- Prosthetic cardiac valves without attached tissue
- Tonsils and adenoids from children*
- Torn meniscus
- Umbilical hernia sacs in children*
- Varicose veins

Revision History
Adopted May 1996
Reaffirmed May 1999
Revised August 1999

* Each institution should determine its own specific age requirements.

Exhibit 3-4. Stewardship of pathologic specimens

College of American Pathologists policy

Policy synopsis

The laboratory that provides the primary evaluation of diagnostic tissues is responsible for the maintenance and integrity of pathology reports, slides, and blocks. That material is held in trust for the patient, creating a fiduciary relationship whereby the pathologist becomes the steward of the material and does not have legal ownership. Appropriate retention periods are determined by CLIA and state regulations. The primary institutional pathologist has a responsibility to safeguard material for the patient's immediate and future needs and must fulfill institutional legal responsibilities related to record keeping and confidentiality. The pathologist's responsibility also includes providing appropriate material for institutionally approved studies with the informed consent of the patient.

Policy

As scientific, medical, economic, and ethical concerns rapidly evolve, pathologists have significant responsibility in fulfilling patient care needs and contributing to advances in medical and scientific knowledge. Institutional and investigative authorities must recognize this responsibility and support the pathologist's role as steward of patient material.

Patient specimens are routinely sent to the pathology laboratory for diagnostic evaluation. All or representative portions of this material are selected and prepared for microscopic evaluation and diagnosis. Paraffin-embedded tissue blocks and the corresponding slides, cytologic smears, and other specimen material then become part of the permanent patient record. Increasingly, such material is subsequently used for additional patient-care related studies such as immunologic and molecular analysis. Materials may also need to be re-evaluated later when new clinical information and/or diagnostic material becomes available. Finally, pathology material (slides and blocks) may be needed for clinicopathologic studies. For these reasons, diagnostic material must remain available in the institution at which it was prepared unless the patient directs their transfer elsewhere. Just as the institution where a patient receives treatment has the responsibility to maintain the medical record, the laboratory that provides the primary evaluation of diagnostic tissues is responsible for the maintenance and integrity of pathology reports, slides, and blocks.

Neither statutory nor case law clearly defines the legal ownership of patient specimens. While the processing of pathology specimens transforms them into durable materials, eg, slides and blocks that may fairly be claimed to be the property of the institution, it is expected that this material will be preserved and protected in a safe and reliable location for the future benefit of the patient. The pathology department, therefore is considered to hold the material in trust for the patient, creating a fiduciary relationship whereby the pathologist becomes the steward of the material and does not have legal ownership, per se. The institution in which the diagnostic material is produced has an obligation to respond to patient needs in terms of future medical care and confidentiality and is therefore the appropriate and logical trustee of this material. When diagnostic material is produced in more than one laboratory, eg, slides, blocks, tissue, or cells sent to another institution for special studies such as immunohistochemistry, electron microscopic, molecular studies, etc, and retained by them, then the consulting laboratories become secondary stewards of the additional material they prepare unless there is an agreement to have such materials retained by the referring institution. Secondary stewards must accept the same responsibility to maintain the integrity of the material.

The appropriate retention period for patient material depends both on the type of material and the disease process identified. Space constraints and technical limitations make the prolonged retention of fixed but unprocessed tissue impractical. The retention of slides and paraffin blocks is a better means of storage and preservation of patient material and their contained medical information. The College of American Pathologists has recommended minimal requirements for the retention of laboratory records and diagnostic materials that meet or exceed the regulatory requirements specified in the Clinical Laboratory Improvement Amendments of 1988 (CLIA '88). Some state regulations may require longer retention periods. Laboratories are encouraged to retain materials for even longer periods of time when patient care needs so warrant.

The responsibility to maintain diagnostic material also includes providing appropriate material for institutionally approved studies when the patient has given informed consent to allow their tissue for research as long as the primary pathology record is not compromised, ie, diagnostic material remains available in the pathology file for future patient care needs. An appropriate balance between patient care needs and investigative studies must be maintained. Although it is not in the patient's best interests for a research group to acquire all of an individual's diagnostic pathology material, patient care usually will not be jeopardized if some material is released for an appropriate study. Determination of the nature and amount of diagnostic pathology material that can be released for research purposes without compromising the medical interests of the patient can best be made by the primary institutional pathologist. This individual is most knowledgeable about the limitations of tissue availability in a given case; has a responsibility to safeguard material for the patient's immediate and future needs; and must fulfill institutional legal responsibilities related to record keeping and confidentiality.

Research based on patient material should not be unduly hindered. Information gained from the study of such material is essential for the advancement of knowledge regarding a disease and/or its treatment. Selected material may be provided for approved research projects if the needs and rights of the patient can be protected. These include the right of appropriate informed consent and privacy as determined by the Institutional Review Board (IRB).[23] Studies that deal with HIV status or possible inherited conditions generally require informed consent when done on samples from identifiable patients. Retrospective studies performed on archived material that has been anonymized and prospectively collected samples that are never linked to a source as defined by current federal regulations require approval of the local IRB. Pathology departments should be fully informed of the current state and federal regulations regarding the use of patient material in research and have a written policy about confidentiality and privacy rights.[24]

Financial concerns are another significant issue related to patient tissues for research. Pathologists and/or the institution should not have to bear the costs incurred in supplying such material. Such costs should be recoverable from the investigator and include those ordinarily associated with specimen retrieval, such as recutting of blocks, special handling, and shipping.

The pathologist must exercise considerable judgment in balancing the many and often conflicting requirements of patient care and scientific advancement. This can only be accomplished through the cooperation of the pathology and research communities, patient advocacy groups, and regulatory agencies.

Revision History
Adopted February 1997
Reaffirmed May 2000

References

1. Medical devices; device tracking. *Fed Reg.* February 8, 2002;67(27):5943-5952. Available at: http://www.fda.gov/cdrh/modact/modernfr.html. Accessed February 4, 2005.

2. Centers for Disease Control and Prevention. Medical examiners, coroners, and biologic terrorism: a guidebook for surveillance and case management. *MMWR.* 2004;53(RR-8):1-36.

3. United States Department of Health & Human Services. Office for Civil Rights - HIPAA. Medical privacy: national standards to protect the privacy of personal health information. Available at: http://www.hhs.gov/ocr/hipaa/. Accessed February 4, 2005.

4. HIPAA Privacy Rule Final Release [special report]. *CAP STATLINE.* August 14, 2002. Available at: http://www.cap.org:80/apps/docs/statline/HIPAA_Special_Report.html. Accessed January 13, 2005.

5. ASCO Working Group. American Society of Clinical Oncology policy statement update: genetic testing for cancer susceptibility. *J Clin Oncol.* 2003; 21(12):1-10.

6. Proposed Genetic Test Standards. CAP STATLINE. March 17, 2004. Available at: http://www.cap.org:80/apps/docs/statline/stat031704.html. Accessed February 4, 2005.

7. Swanson PE. Labels, disclaimers, and rules (oh, my!). *Am J Clin Pathol.* 1999;111:445-448.

8. Taylor CR. FDA issues final rule for classification/reclassification of immunochemistry reagents and kits [editorial]. *Appl Immunohistochem.* 1998;6:115-116.

9. Sentinel events. In: *Joint Commission on Accreditation of Healthcare Organizations. 2004 and 2005 Comprehensive Accreditation Manual for Hospital: The Official Handbook (CAMH).* Available at: http://www.jcrinc.com/subscribers/perspectives.asp?durki=6065&site= 10&return=2815. Accessed February 4, 2005.

10. Wakely SL, Baxendine-Jones JA, Gallagher PJ, Mullee M, Pickering R. Aberrant diagnoses by individual surgical pathologists. *Am J Surg Pathol.* 1998;22:77-82.

11. Zarbo RJ, Nakhleh RE. Surgical pathology specimens for gross examination only and exempt from submission: a College of American Pathologists Q-Probes study of current policies in 413 institutions. *Arch Pathol Lab Med.* 1999;123:133-139.

12. Fitzgibbons PL, Cleary K. CAP recommendations on submission of specimens to pathology. *CAP Today.* 1996;10(7):40.

13. Association of Directors of Anatomic and Surgical Pathology. Consultations in surgical pathology. *Am J Surg Pathol.* 1993;17:743-745.

14. Cooper K, Fitzgibbons PL. Institutional consultations in surgical pathology: how should diagnostic disagreements be handled? *Arch Pathol Lab Med.* 2002;126:650-651.

15. Swisher BL, Ewing EP. Frozen section technique for tissues infected by the AIDS virus. *J Histotechnol.* 1986;9:29.

16. Nakhleh R, Zarbo RJ. Amended reports in surgical pathology and implication for diagnostic error detection and avoidance: a College of American Pathologists Q-Probes study of 1,667,547 accessioned cases in 359 laboratories. *Arch Pathol Lab Med.* 1998;122:303-309.

17. Merrick TA, Carter DK. Patient requests for gallstones [Q&A]. *CAP Today.* September 2002.

18. Fitzgibbons PL, LiVolsi VA. Surgical Pathology Committee of the College of American Pathologists, Association of Directors of Anatomic Surgical Pathology. Recommendations for handling radioactive specimens obtained by sentinel lymphadenectomy. *Am J Surg Pathol.* 2000;24:1549-1551.

19. Fitzgibbons PL. Retention of silicone breast prostheses [Q&A]. *CAP Today.* July 2004:142.

20. Borkowski A, Lee DH, Sydnor DL, et al. Intranet-based quality improvement documentation at the Veterans Affairs Maryland Health Care System. *Mod Pathol.* 2001;14:1-5.

21. Althshuler G, Deppisch LM. CAP Conference XIX on the examination of the placenta: report of the working group on indications for placental examination. *Arch Pathol Lab Med.* 1991;115:701-703.

22. Revised CAP guidelines for prosthetic breast implants. *CAP Today.* April 95;Vol. 9:58.

23. Pathology Consensus Statement: Uses of Human Tissue. August 28, 1996.

24. Grizzle W, Grody WW, Noll WW, et al. Recommended policies for uses of human tissue in research, education and quality control. *Arch Pathol Lab Med.* 1999;123:296-300.

Bibliography

American Society of Clinical Oncology. Policy statement update: genetic testing for cancer susceptibility. *J Clin Oncol.* 2003;21(12):1-10.

Bioterrorism: A Special Report. *CAP STATLINE.* August 14, 2002. Available at http://www.cap.org:80/apps/docs/statline/statbio.html. Accessed January 13, 2005.

Merrick TA. Cryostat disinfection [Q&A]. *CAP Today.* May 2004:93.

Mohapatra S, Kalogjera L. Who owns these slides?: overview of legal issues facing pathologists and laboratories when saving and sending out tissues, slides, and tissue blocks. *Pathol Case Rev.* 2003;8(3):90-97.

Pereira TC, Liu Y, Silverman JF. Critical values in surgical pathology. *Am J Clin Pathol.* 2004; 122:201-205.

Recommendations to CAP Membership on Mercury Reduction. DRAFT of Working Group of CAP Council on Scientific Affairs. July 2004.

Travers H. HIPAA privacy regulations [Q&A]. *CAP Today.* February 2003.

Yost JA. Laboratory inspection: the view from CMS. *Lab Med.* 2003;34(2):136-40.

Zarbo RJ, Nakhleh RE, Walsh M, Quality Practices Committee, College of American Pathologists. Customer satisfaction in anatomic pathology: a College of American Pathologists Q-Probes study of 3065 physician surveys from 94 laboratories. *Arch Pathol Lab Med.* 2003;127(1):23-9.

Strategies for error reduction and prevention in surgical pathology

Raouf E. Nakhleh, MD

Surgical pathology is an inherently complex system that depends on a multitude of individuals (inside and outside the laboratory) to do their jobs well and deliver an error-free report. Total automation represents the ultimate solution to error reduction, whereby a specimen is identified by the patient's DNA and is placed in a machine, where it is dissected, processed, and slides are made. The slides are then interpreted and a computer-based report is generated, which includes complete clinical information and differential diagnoses, with decision pathways tied to ancillary studies. The system would challenge or reject incomplete reports and those with nonsensical answers. Although such a machine is not yet available, a clear path is charted for the future when automation increasingly will be used to improve specimen identification and processing methods, and computer aids will support diagnoses and complete pathology reports.

While errors occur for many reasons, factors that contribute to system failure and errors include variable input, complexity, inconsistency, tight coupling, human intervention, time constraints, and an inflexible hierarchical culture.

- Varied input leads to errors because the system has to be modified to accommodate the input. By contrast, uniform input leads to consistent processes and uniform output.

- System complexity increases the chance of error. It has been estimated that if each step in a process has a 1% chance of error, 25 steps will increase the chance of error to 22%. With 50 steps, the chance grows to 39%.

- Inconsistencies at any level leads to errors and may be seen in training, individual performance, procedures, or communication, including diagnostic language or taxonomy.

- When steps are tightly coupled, there is no room to recognize and deal with variation. The result may be akin to forcing a square peg into a round hole.

- Human intervention is more prone to error in routine tasks. This contrasts with machines, which can accomplish routine tasks better than humans but don't do as well when things go wrong. Human judgment is still superior to machines when unanticipated conditions arise.

- Tight time constraints lead to tight coupling between steps, reducing the opportunity to identify and handle variations. Very loose time constraints can also lead to failures, possibly due to boredom or distraction.

- A group of individuals working as a team where communication is not constrained by rank or job will function better than a group that is constrained by hierarchical conventions.

In this chapter, we offer information on general principles of error reduction along with specific methods in surgical pathology that have been shown to reduce errors. Error reduction, unfortunately, cannot simply be turned on with the implementation of one of these methods.

Sustained error reduction only comes with a persistent effort to address all aspects of the laboratory with good monitoring tools to evaluate how well a system functions.

General principles of error reduction

Broad principles of error reduction may be divided into the following general categories: (1) system solutions, or those related to the structure and function of work processes; and (2) personnel solutions, related to having the right people doing the job at the right time.

System solutions

Reduce reliance on memory

Continuously relying on memory to do complex tasks ultimately leads to mistakes. As much as possible, introduce memory aids into systems. These may include using checklists and protocols to accomplish daily tasks ranging from quality control functions to daily work logs.

Examples of memory aides include computerized synoptic checklists, used to assure that cancer reports are complete. Although automated equipment for routine, special, and immunohistochemistry stains are not thought of as memory aids, they do alleviate the need to remember complex multi-step procedures. In general, automation reduces reliance on memory.

Reducing reliance on memory helps address the problems of variable input, complexity, inconsistency, and human intervention.

Improve information access

Display information where and when it is needed, in a form that permits easy access to those who need it. Access to clinical information is most helpful at the time of slide interpretation. During frozen section evaluation, a full understanding of the patient's history, including radiographic and previous pathologic diagnosis, can facilitate the pathologist's attention to the clinical question at hand, such as margins or extent of disease, rather than diverting attention to diagnostic dilemmas.

Having access to an electronic medical record is equally important during final sign-out. Such access facilitates one's ability to get information, saves time, and facilitates clinical correlation with other studies or previous pathologic diagnoses.

Improved information access addresses concerns of variable input and inconsistency.

Error-proof processes: use constraints and forcing functions

This mechanism of error reduction attempts to control an operation by reducing the number of options and, in essence, to automate a process to completion. This works well with tasks such as specimen accessioning. When a case is accessioned, the computer system forces the check of the patient's identity by using a name and a second unique identifier, and checking for prior accessions against other information previously entered into the system. A number of other information items may be required before accessioning is done, including specimen type, ICD-9 codes, and billing codes. This provides for uniform input of patient information.

In a comprehensive system, the case number is generated and is automatically added to case logs for histology, the pathologist, and transcription. In addition, if block and slide labeling machines are used, the blocks and slides may be printed automatically without the need to rewrite the accession number. Furthermore, depending on the type of specimen, the number of levels, and the need for any specific stains or other studies, orders may be automatically generated for histology.

In a system with such cascading effects, serious problems can arise when the initial step is not done correctly. Workers must be trained to recognize and investigate problems before accessioning, and not attempt to force cases through the system. Clear instructions must be outlined on how to deal with unfamiliar situations.

The use of constraints and forcing function is an attempt to address complexity.

Decrease reliance on vigilance

Many laboratories depend on the vigilance of key individuals to avoid error. While it is desirable to have excellent workers who care deeply for their work, the laboratory cannot be totally dependent on human vigilance. A system needs to be built with internal checks and clear logical pathways for all to follow.

A comprehensive computer system is very helpful in producing internal checks on all processes within a system. For example, if remote order entry is available, the laboratory has advance notice of an incoming specimen. As accessioning proceeds, the computer system at specified times will generate a list of cases that have not yet been received, leading to inquiries as to the specimen's location.

Bar codes are a great aid to input cases at each step, including accessioning, grossing, microscopic dictation, and transcription. This reduces input errors, although one must be vigilant to scan the right case. This also provides for tracking specimens as they are processed through the lab and generating work logs. While checking these case logs may be referred to as vigilance, these checks work best when they are integrated into the daily routine rather than trusting that the work is done.

Reducing reliance on vigilance helps address variable input, problems of human intervention, and complexity.

Standardize tasks and language

To reduce errors, it is best to standardize all procedures relevant to the laboratory. This extends from policies and procedures related to specimen procurement and acceptability, to distribution of pathology reports. Having one method reduces errors in two ways. First, reducing competing methodologies and ensuring consistency simplify training. Second, reduced variation in methods reduces errors by reducing guesswork about which method to use.

Standardizing language is just as important. This applies to the use of language within the laboratory to reduce confusion, such as distinguishing the difference between a recut and a level. Perhaps more important is the standardization of diagnostic language across institutions. This is a lofty goal—one that is difficult to achieve quickly. The College of American Pathologists and the American College of Surgeons have together taken a leadership role in standardizing cancer terminology by developing and implementing standardized data reporting elements. Most important is the need for pathologists to standardize diagnostic language with clinicians of the same institution.

Standardizing tasks and language addresses problems of human intervention, variable input, complexity and inconsistency.

Reduce the number of hand-offs: simplify the process

Hand-offs are focal points for errors. There are multiple hand-offs in surgical pathology, starting with specimen collection in the clinician's office or surgical suite. After acceptance in the laboratory at accessioning, the specimen is handed off for grossing, then to histology, where the specimen is transferred from the block to the slide, and then to the pathologist, who subsequently hands it off to transcription. The case is then verified and handed back to the clinician.

Ideally, reducing the number of hand-offs and error-proofing the hand-offs would reduce errors. Unfortunately, no machine has been invented to remove these hand-offs. However, some technologic and other advances have been made that can error-proof these hand-offs, including:

- Remote order entry, with specimen logs to track specimens
- Accessioning with two ID's and access to medical records
- Using bar code technology on protocols and reports, and hopefully soon, on slides and blocks
- Tying accessioning with block and slide labeling
- Removing distraction from hand-off areas

Reducing the number of hand-offs addresses complexity.

Design for errors

Design a system that encourages error detection and correction before a problem occurs. This means a system should be built with many quality assurance and quality control monitors incorporated into daily functions. Specimen logs at each step are important to assure that every specimen is accounted for in real time. This may also include a double-check on error-prone areas, such as a mandatory second opinion on selected cases.

Designing for errors helps address problems of tight coupling, time constraints, variable input, and inconsistencies.

Personnel solutions

Adjust work schedules

Many errors occur during times of stress. The laboratory director and the laboratory supervisor must have a good understanding of the workflow, particularly when the amount of work is greatest. There is a clear need to understand the number of people needed to accomplish a required task in a timely fashion. At the same time, schedules must be balanced so that tasks not constrained by time may be accomplished during slower periods.

Reducing errors requires emphasizing doing a job correctly rather than quickly. It is management's duty to make sure that enough people are available to do the job in a timely and accurate manner.

Adjusting work schedules primarily addresses time constraints.

Adjust the environment

There are basic requirements for the physical environment, such as adequate space. Errors occur more easily when specimens are piled up on a counter for grossing such that the wrong specimen or cassette may be picked up. A similar situation may occur at the time of slide preparation in histology. Other physical conditions, such as lighting and the general feel of the lab, are important in conveying a pleasant physical environment.

The psychological environment is equally as important. Workers are most productive in a nurturing professional environment with clearly understood responsibilities. An environment of blame and shame is destructive and ultimately leads to self-protective behavior, which is counterproductive to reducing error.

Adjusting the environment is an attempt to address problems with time constraints and a hierarchical culture.

Provide adequate training

While job qualifications are defined and in some states even regulated, an individual must be trained to do their job within the parameters and systems of a particular laboratory. Individuals must be trained without ambiguity to understand their responsibilities in a broad sense and, where applicable, regarding specific tasks. There should be no guesswork. Training should be verified by a period of observation, followed by periodic review. Training must also be provided for safety and quality improvement.

Training addresses many problems, including those of inconsistency, human intervention, tight time constraints, and a hierarchical culture.

Choose the right staff for the job

While multiple individuals may meet basic qualifications for a job, it is clear that individuals vary in their strengths and weaknesses. Having a group of individuals with complementary strengths, but with adequate redundancy in vital areas, is key to having a functioning productive laboratory. This applies to all groups within surgical pathology, including pathologists, pathologist assistants, histotechnologists, secretaries, and other support personal.

Appropriate staffing addresses problems of human intervention and a hierarchical culture.

Methods that may reduce errors in surgical pathology

Below is a list of specific interventions that have been suggested from numerous resources, which may be helpful in reducing errors. Please note that some of these interventions may not be effective or applicable to your particular laboratory.

Entire test cycle

- Utilize a fully-integrated computer system

- Build in quality assurance and quality control steps

- Establish and maintain good communication

- Provide adequate staffing

- Ensure the right people are doing the right job

- Minimize distractions, particularly at accessioning, gross examination, slide cutting, slide interpretation, transcription, and report verification

Preanalytic phase: specimen delivery and accessioning

- Use remote order entry or other tracking mechanism

- Establish clear responsibility for delivery of the specimen to the laboratory

- Agree on pick-up and delivery time for optimal processing

- Provide proper storage and delivery containers

- Adhere to strict labeling standards, with clear guidelines for handling improperly labeled specimens

- Maintain good guidelines for specimen procurement and fixation, with easily found references

- Establish clear specimen acceptability standards, with clear directions on how to deal with unacceptable specimens

- Use accessioning systems that correlate with previous accessions and the patients' medical record

- Provide clear instructions on how to assure proper identification of specimens during accessioning

- Avoid sequential accessioning of similar specimens

- Accession sequential cases with different color cassettes matched with protocol labels and slides, as has been suggested by some

- Eliminate distractions when accessioning by ensuring that employees do not have other duties

Analytic phase: technical factors

- Reduce the stress level

- Reduce the feeling of being rushed—emphasize safety over speed

- Practice within your area of expertise

- Seek help when you feel uncomfortable

- Provide and ensure proper training for handling different situations

- Obtain consensus on taxonomy and methodology

- Use appropriate specimen wraps or bags

- Clean instruments and cutting board between gross room cases

- Change gloves between large gross-room cases

- Take care not to introduce or pick up floaters when using a cryobath

- Label frozen section slides with two identifiers

- Confirm the patient's ID when reporting a frozen section

- Keep separate any concurrent frozen section cases

- Take appropriate size sections for optimal fixation and processing

- Use automatic block and slide labelers, if possible

- Inspect machine settings daily

- Replace or fill instrument reagents according to specifications

- Maintain instruments in good operating condition

- Use end-of-day checklist to assure proper fixation and processing of tissues

- Use bar codes, where possible, with scanners (requisition slip, specimen container, blocks, slides, and protocols)

- Minimize distractions at gross examination

- Use two identifiers throughout the process, even on blocks and slides

- Use checklists in the gross room for some specimens

- Match slides with blocks

- Have only the slides for a particular block available while that block is being cut

- Eliminate distraction, such as phone calls, while an employee is cutting

- Match slides with protocol gross dictations (number and gross appearance)

- Put space between different cases on a slide tray

- Put similar cases on different slide trays

- Confirm case number for special stains and recuts with patient name

Analytic phase: diagnostic factors

- Reduce the stress level

- Reduce the feeling of being rushed—emphasize safety over speed

- Practice within your area of expertise

- Seek help when you feel uncomfortable

- Define for the group any specimen that should have a second opinion

- Use checklists for cancer cases and possibly others

- Maintain easy access to the patient's medical record

- Seek additional information whenever necessary

- Correlate findings with the clinical history

- Minimize distractions at slide interpretation and report verification

Postanalytic phase: transcription

- Reduce the stress level

- Reduce the feeling of being rushed—emphasize safety over speed

- Double-check transcribed items against the requisition slip

- Proofread all documents

- Double-check specimen site (especially right and left) against the specimen request slip

- Verbally check with the pathologist assistants or pathologists when something does not make sense

- Maintain and use case logs to track outstanding cases from accessioning to report finalization

- Use case logs to assure that all cases are finalized

Bibliography

1. Cohen MM, Eustis MA, Gribbins RE. Changing the culture of patient safety: leadership's role in health care quality improvement. *Jt Comm J Qual Saf.* 2003;29:329-335.
2. Grout JR. Preventing medical errors by designing benign failures. *Jt Comm J Qual Saf.* 2003;29:354-362.
3. Petersen D. Human *Error Reduction and Safety Management.* 3rd ed. New York: International Thomson Publishing Inc; 1996.
4. Spath PL, ed. *Error Reduction in Health Care: A Systems Approach to Improving Patient Safety.* San Francisco, Calif: Jossey-Bass Publishers; 2000.
5. Welch DL. Human error and human factor engineering in health care. *Biomed Instrum Technol.* 1997;31;627-631.

Defining and handling errors in surgical pathology

John E. Tomaszewski, MD
Virginia A. LiVolsi, MD

There are no measures of surgical pathology performance that are currently mandated by law, and relatively few that are recommended by accrediting agencies. This is not because performance is unimportant, but because of the difficulty in determining how it should be defined and measured. For example, after more than 10 years of legally mandated review of Pap smear interpretation, there remains no consensus on the best way to assess the performance of this test or what typical laboratory results should be.[1] Defining and measuring performance in surgical pathology is even more complex, and there have been few comprehensive studies on this subject. Nonetheless, pressure from clinicians, patients, regulators, and payers underscores an increasing interest in documenting acceptable performance in surgical pathology. Pathologists are also interested in such measures as a means to identify areas for quality improvement.

Because of the wide variety of neoplastic and non-neoplastic lesions that must be considered, and because many cases require evaluation of multiple elements, an unequivocal gold standard for test accuracy rarely exists in surgical pathology. Accurately measuring surgical pathology performance, ie, the "correctness" of the diagnosis, ideally involves correlating the diagnosis with all other pertinent clinical information and patient outcome. However, such a complex performance measuring system is impractical for daily operational needs, and other approaches have been adopted. Unfortunately, most current quality assurance programs do not measure performance directly, but instead identify problems (ie, a lack of performance).

Despite its reliance on individual (subjective) opinion, peer review has become an important method of evaluating diagnostic accuracy. In surgical pathology, the frequency of diagnostic differences on second opinion slide review varies widely in the literature, ranging from 0.5% to 43%. Diagnostic disagreements that are associated with medical "significance" are also reported to occupy a wide range,[1] with published values from 0.25% to 24%. A great deal of variability also is reported among specific organ systems. Reported diagnostic accuracy rates are lowest for neuropathology,[2-4] gynecological pathology,[5] sarcomas,[6] and specimens from cytology cases and serosal surfaces.[7]

Renshaw[1] has divided errors into the following categories:

- **False-negative** (diagnosis made on second review that was not made initially)
- **False-positive** (diagnosis that the reviewer thought was not present)
- **Threshold** (difference of opinion relating to a diagnostic threshold)
- **Type and grade** (differences in tumor typing and grading)
- **Missed margin** (positive margins that are missed)
- **Other**

In this schema, the most frequent type of error in studies reviewing consecutive cases was false-negative error. By contrast, in series that were based on selected consultation cases, the most frequent types of error were false-positive, threshold, and type and grade errors. Intraoperative consultations generate a special form of re-review, comparing the diagnoses produced from two standard but differing histopathological techniques. The frequency of discrepancies between frozen sections and permanent sections in a large interinstitutional survey[8] is 1.7%.

Mechanisms for discovery of error

Error may be discovered during routine clinical work as part of historic case query and review procedures (eg, 5-year look back for gynecologic cytology), or it may be discovered in the context of an institution's quality improvement program. In each instance, the error may be chronologically proximate or distant to the index pathological exam.

There are a number of review mechanisms by which a quality assurance program can detect errors. These include but are not limited to the following:

- Intraoperative consultation review (frozen section/permanent section correlation)
- Intradepartmental quality assurance conferences
- Review of prior cytology or surgical (historic) material
- Random case review
- Topic directed periodic reviews
- Intradepartmental review prior to release of materials to an outside institution
- Interdepartmental conferences (eg, tumor boards)

Each of these mechanisms offers a unique opportunity to discover problems and improve performance at different times in the patient care sequence. In general, quality assurance mechanisms that discover error proximate to index events are most valuable.

Review of historic material is often precipitated by the need for morphological comparison to accurately interpret a current specimen but may also be a component of a quality assurance program.

Definitions of diagnostic discrepancies

Traditionally, diagnostic discrepancies have been divided into major and minor categories, as defined below.

Major discrepancies are those that fulfill two criteria. The discrepancy must represent a significant change between the original diagnosis and the one rendered upon review, and the discrepancy must potentially have a serious impact on the patient's treatment or prognosis. Examples include reversal of a benign diagnosis to malignant, reversal of a malignant diagnosis to benign, and failure to recognize a specific treatable inflammatory condition (eg, infectious organism).

Minor discrepancies are those in which a small change in diagnosis is found, but there is minimal, if any, clinical relevance. Examples include changes in tumor grade or misclassification of a neoplasm (eg, follicular variant of papillary thyroid carcinoma interpreted as follicular carcinoma).

However, an identical discrepancy or error may lead to vastly different consequences, depending on the timing of error discovery and the actions taken by the clinician. For this reason, the classification of discrepancies is best done in a more objective fashion, as described by Renshaw[1] (ie, false-positive, false-negative, problem of threshold, problem of type and grade, missed margin or other). This, however, should be tempered and actions taken based on the likely impact to the patient. Impact on patient care is usually classified as significant, slight, or no impact to patient care. In addition, many institutions will classify how the error or discrepancy may have occurred (clerical, misidentification or labeling errors, lack of clinical information or correlation, gross or microscopic sampling, technical problems, and misinterpretation).

This classification scheme allows for more objective data while keeping the focus on patient care. Therefore errors and discrepancies of all types can be addressed in a systematic fashion, and system modifications may be implemented in a more directed fashion to effect change and reduce errors.

Relative risks by time of discovery

Errors may have different clinical and therapeutic consequences depending upon the temporal relationship between the initial diagnosis and the identification of a diagnostic discrepancy. We have divided these into the following three categories.

Nearly immediate identification of discrepancy

Temporally, this usually implies no more than a few days from the time the original report was issued. If mistakes are uncovered within a short period of time, errors can be corrected before therapy is instituted. The risk to the physical health of the patient in such cases should be minimal.

A subset of these errors includes those in which a frozen section diagnosis is reversed when permanent control sections are examined. In this case, significant surgery or other major intraoperative intervention may have occurred based on the initial frozen section diagnosis. Communication with the treating physician (preferably verbally and in writing) is mandated; the final pathology report must resolve the discrepancy between the initial frozen section interpretation and the final diagnosis.

Intermediate time to identification of discrepancy

These discrepancies often are discovered when slides are sent for patient-requested or clinician-requested second opinion and may be identified by reviewing the slides before they are released or by a pathologist at another institution. It may be difficult to assess whether or not treatment has been instituted, but second opinions often are obtained before definitive therapy has begun. Hence, physical harm to the patient because of pathological misinterpretation may not have occurred. Pathologic review of all outside cases before surgery or the initiation of therapy may decrease the potential for harm from such discrepancies.

Extended time to identification of discrepancy

These discrepancies are identified late in the patient's clinical course, sometimes after treatment has been completed. In these instances, review of slides from an earlier biopsy or resection (often months or even years prior to examination of the current specimen) discloses a major reversal in diagnosis. Often this involves an underdiagnosis of malignancy.

Response to error discovery

The response to error discovery must follow established policies within the institution. All pathology departments should maintain a description of the steps followed when significant errors are discovered, which may include notifying the hospital's risk management department, the departmental chair (when appropriate), and the institutional quality practices committee.

Responses to the discovery of serious errors should adhere to these established policies:

- Errors or discrepancies that may have a significant impact on patient care must be reported to the responsible clinician(s). If a change in care will result from this discovery, a revised or corrected pathology report (as defined previously) should be issued. Determining the circumstances by which the patient is notified is made in conjunction with the responsible clinician(s).

- Errors or discrepancies with no impact on patient care should be forwarded to the departmental quality assurance program for analysis, as accumulated data may suggest practice pattern improvements.

- Errors discovered very near the time of the original pathology report are usually handled by issuing a corrected, revised, or addendum report and notifying the responsible clinician(s).

- The response to a diagnostic discrepancy detected late in the patient's clinical course may vary depending upon the nature of the error and likely impact on the clinical care of the patient. Errors that may impact the patient's care should be referred to the appropriate institutional committee for evaluation, possible action, and root cause analysis.

Summary

While there are multiple ways errors and discrepancies come to light, the appropriate response is largely dependent upon where they fall in a two-by-three matrix defined by the potential for patient harm (significant versus minimal) and the timeliness of discovery (short, intermediate, long). An effective quality improvement program in anatomic pathology should result in a decreased proportion of all errors discovered after a significant time interval. Critically assessing these trends can allow one to evaluate the effectiveness of the program.

References

1. Renshaw AA. Measuring and reporting errors in surgical pathology. *Am J Clin Pathol.* 2001;115:338-341.
2. Bruner JM, Inouye L, Fuller GN, et al. Diagnostic discrepancies and their clinical impact in a neuropathology referral practice. *Cancer.* 1997;79:796-803.
3. Scott CB, Nelson JS, Farnan NC, et al. Central pathology review in clinical trials for patients with malignant glioma. *Cancer.* 1995;76:307-313.
4. Aldape K, Simmons ML, Davis RL, et al. Discrepancies in diagnoses of neuroepithelial neoplasms: The San Francisco Bay Area Adult Glioma Study. *Cancer.* 2000;88:2342-2349.
5. Selman AE, Niemann TH, Fowler JM, et al. Quality assurance of second opinion in gynecologic oncology. *Obstet Gynecol.* 1999;94:302-306.
6. Harris M, Hartley AL, Blair V, et al. Sarcomas in northwest England, I: histopathological peer review. *Br J Cancer.* 1991;64:315-320.
7. Kronz JD, Westra WH, Epstein JI. Mandatory second opinion surgical pathology at a large referral hospital. *Cancer.* 1999;86:2426-2438.
8. Zarbo RJ, Hoffman GG, Howanitz PJ. Interinstitutional comparison of frozen-section consultation: a College of American Pathologists Q-Probes study of 79,647 consultations in 297 North American institutions. *Arch Pathol Lab Med.* 1991;115:1187-1194.

Quality improvement plan components and monitors

Overview

A continuous quality improvement (CQI) plan generates data that can be used to identify problems and recognize opportunities for improvement. Besides identifying trends, a quality assurance program should also detect medical errors and provide data that can be used to improve patient safety. The starting point for monitoring and evaluation is the development of appropriate indicators (measurable variables) to audit the most important aspects of care provided.

Each quality indicator (monitor) should have a defined method of data collection and organization. The data are then analyzed and interpreted to identify potential or actual problems uncovered by this monitoring process. In order to put the interpretation of raw numbers or results into an appropriate context, benchmarks or standards of practice should be established for each activity. Threshold limits for indicators should be defined using an institutional database or, preferably, incorporating interinstitutional peer group comparisons when possible. Thresholds help set realistic goals for improvement and create a rational basis for action, which may include a focused audit. Serious deviations or "sentinel events" automatically require in-depth review and should always have an expected compliance threshold of 100%

Preanalytic variables: specimen submission and handling

Richard W. Brown, MD

Background

Each institution should have a set of guidelines for submitting tissues and other specimens to the surgical pathology laboratory. These guidelines should be clearly defined in a written manual available at all submitting sites and should include:

- Types of specimens to be submitted and those excluded from pathologic examination (see chapter 3, Exhibit 3-3)
- Preferred mode of submission (eg, fresh, fixed) and, if the latter, special fixation requirements
- Instructions for completing the surgical pathology requisition form
- Criteria used by the laboratory for specimen rejection

Specimen procurement encompasses all activities from the removal of the specimen to its acceptance by the pathology laboratory. Accordingly, this process requires close cooperation and communication between the surgeon, the operating room nursing and technical staff, the clerical and technical staff of the surgical pathology laboratory, and the pathologist. For specimens obtained outside the operating rooms or hospital, established procedures should be rigorously followed since communication among those involved usually is more difficult.

Specimen procurement, transport, and accessioning

The procurement of specimens for histologic evaluation consists of the following elements:

■ Correct identification and integrity of identification (labeling)
■ A properly completed surgical pathology requisition
■ Fixation and handling appropriate for the specimen
■ Prompt delivery of the specimen to the laboratory
■ Proper accessioning

The submitting physician has responsibility for initial specimen handling, including preservation and labeling. Specimen transportation typically is provided by the institution (OR nurses, runners, etc) and is often not under direct control of laboratory personnel. While the pathology department may not be responsible for specimens until they are accepted in the laboratory, pathologists should actively promote cooperative mechanisms with other departments to ensure optimum specimen handling.

Correct identification of submitted specimens

A surgical pathology specimen is typically the result of an invasive procedure and often includes a lesion in its entirety. Therefore correct identification and integrity of identification, from specimen removal to accessioning within the laboratory, are essential. Proper identification must be on the container and should include at least:

■ Patient's full name
■ Unique identifying number
■ Sex
■ Age (date of birth)
■ Date obtained
■ Organ/tissue site

This identifying information must match the information on the specimen requisition form (see next section). In general, the identification should be placed on the body of the container holding the specimen rather than on the lid, which may be inadvertently transferred. Standard safety precautions should be followed in handling all specimens; however, if a specimen presents a known or suspected biohazard, the container should be so marked.

The person who accessions the specimen into the surgical pathology laboratory should not accept specimens that are improperly labeled, incompletely labeled, or lack an accompanying specimen requisition in strict accordance with the department's procedures for specimen submission. However, due to the uniqueness of most surgical pathology specimens, rejection should not occur until an exhaustive attempt has been made to correct the deficiency.

Data collection

A specimen "rejection" log should be maintained to document all cases in which deficiencies are identified; a suggested format is provided in Table 6-1. All changes to specimen labels or requisitions should be initialed and dated by the correcting personnel. Depending on institutional policy, it may be useful to further document in the rejection log, or in a separate incident report, the names of the personnel involved and the time elapsed from initial contact to final resolution. Periodic review of

Table 6-1. Specimen rejection log

Date	Patient	Clinic/Location	Reason for Rejection*	Action Taken
2/05/2005	ABC	OR 17	No accompanying requisition form	Surgery staff contacted; requisition received
2/11/2005	DEF	Dermatology clinic	Identification on specimen container does not match requisition	Surgery staff contacted; specimen properly identified
3/05/2005	GHI	GYN clinic	Third portion of specimen not received	Surgery staff contacted; specimen located in operating room

* Coded data entry may be used to allow for easy categorization of deficiency.

this data should be done, with emphasis on the rate of deficiencies and special attention given to problematic locations or recurrent deficiencies.

Benchmark data

A 1994 Q-Probes study,[1] involving 1,004,115 cases from 417 institutions, documented identification and accessioning deficiencies in 6% of total cases accessioned, with a median deficiency rate of 3.4%. Errors related to specimen identification accounted for 9.6% of these deficiencies, discrepant or missing information items were present in 77%, and 3.6% involved specimen handling.

In this same report, it was noted that deficiencies in specimen identification were most frequently resolved by telephone or fax transmissions (25.3%), direct identification/correction by the Submitting nurse (10.6%), or by returning the specimen (8.7%). Notably, in only 0.5% of cases did failure to resolve the problem result in specimen rejection.

Requisition form

Background

A properly completed requisition form should include the following:

- Patient's full name
- Unique identifying number (Social Security number, medical record number, etc)
- Sex and date of birth
- Name of submitting physician (and other pertinent clinicians)
- Date of specimen collection
- Site of specimen
- Brief clinical history
- Preoperative and/or postoperative diagnosis

A requisition form must accompany all specimens, and all identifying information on the requisition must match that on the specimen container(s). If a specimen presents a known or suspected biohazard, this information should be included on the requisition form. Laboratory

Table 6-2. Requisition form monitor

Case No.	Date	Patient Information	Source of Tissue	Clinical History	Submitting Physician
05-2001					
05-2002					
05-2003					
05-2004					
05-2005					

personnel should regularly communicate to the operating room staff the critical nature of proper patient identification. Institutional policies should be in place to ensure that the patient identification information submitted to the laboratory is rigorously compared to the patient's wristband in a manner analogous to that used for blood transfusion.

Data collection

At least quarterly (or more often, depending on the number of specimens received), a subset of the requisitions should be reviewed for completeness. The mechanism of this review should be determined by, and documented in, a written departmental policy. A sample form in checklist format is shown in Table 6-2. Results should be incorporated into departmental and institutional quality reviews, and problems with individual physicians or submission sites should be addressed with the responsible personnel.

Benchmark data

Failure to provide adequate clinical history is a common problem, comprising 40.4% of all deficiencies noted in the 1994 Q-Probes study of specimen identification and accessioning.[1] In monitoring specimen requisitions, a department must determine whether "adequate" is defined as completion of all appropriate fields in the requisition or the presence of sufficient information for informed pathologic diagnosis. A 1996 Q-Probes study of 771,475 surgical pathology cases from 341 institutions found that only 0.73% of cases required additional information before a diagnosis could be rendered.[2] In that study, however, cases that had no clinical information on the requisition slip were not counted if the lack of history did not prevent the rendering of a diagnosis.

Fixation

Background

Specimens may be submitted without fixative if they are delivered to the surgical pathology laboratory promptly and/or if adequate facilities for specimen refrigeration are available. When routine specimen fixation is required by laboratory policy, the appropriate fixative for each specimen type must be designated in the specimen submission manual, and these fixatives should be made readily available. Exceptions to routine fixation, particularly frozen sections and cases with suspected infection or lymphoma, should be carefully emphasized with operating room and laboratory staff.

Table 6-3. Adequacy and appropriateness of fixation

Date	Patient Name/ Accession Number	Problem	Follow-up
1/09/05	ABC	Specimen for frozen section received in formalin	Operating room personnel instructed regarding appropriate procedure
2/16/05	DEF	Biopsy specimen received in saline	Formalin-filled specimen bottles supplied to physician's office
3/20/05	GHI	Large colon resection received in minimal formalin	Operating room personnel instructed regarding amount of fixative required
4/28/05	XYZ	Renal biopsy for glomerular disease received in formalin	Vials with premeasured IF and EM fixatives provided to radiology with instructions for use

In some cases, reviewing the operative schedule and contacting the operating room in advance to communicate specific specimen submission requirements may be appropriate.

Data collection

Specimen submission in an improper fixative or inadequate amounts of fixative should be documented as shown in Table 6-3. Depending on institutional policy, it may be useful to further document in this log, or in a separate incident report, the personnel involved and whether specimen integrity or ability to render a diagnosis was compromised.

Timeliness of delivery to the laboratory

In general, specimens should be delivered to the laboratory as soon as they are obtained. Checking specimens received against those expected by reviewing the daily surgical schedule is often useful. When anticipated specimens are not received, prompt inquiry can be initiated to avoid lost, mishandled, or misplaced specimens. As an additional safeguard, it is advisable to have in place a laboratory policy in which all sections of the laboratory, particularly microbiology, are instructed to notify the surgical pathology laboratory immediately when tissue is received, in order to confirm that a separate specimen was submitted for histologic examination. If problems with timely specimen delivery are encountered, a routine quality assurance monitor should be instituted; this can be easily accomplished by time stamping the requisition at the site of origin and on arrival at the pathology laboratory, and calculating the time elapsed. Individual events resulting in diagnostic delay or compromise in specimen integrity should be documented in a departmental exceptions log and/or incident report as previously described.

Analytic variables: diagnostic accuracy

Mark A. Weiss, MD

Correlation of intraoperative and final diagnoses

Background

Monitoring the correlation of intraoperative and final diagnoses is an integral component of the quality assurance/quality improvement program. It provides a measure of individual and group performance with respect to intraoperative diagnostic accuracy and is important when analyzing outcomes. The review should be a continuous process that includes all cases submitted for intraoperative consultation, including those in which a frozen section (FS) is not performed. The intraoperative decision not to perform a frozen section is as critical as rendering a diagnosis on a frozen section slide, and appropriateness and accuracy of these determinations should also be evaluated.

The Association of Directors of Anatomic and Surgical Pathology (ADASP) has recommended the following correlation categories[3]:

- Agreement
- Deferral – Appropriate
- Deferral – Inappropriate
- Disagreement – Minor
- Disagreement – Major

Each frozen section discordance should be treated as a sentinel event that requires investigation and action, and discrepancies should be reconciled in the final pathology report (CAP Laboratory Accreditation Program checklist item ANP.10100). Determining the reasons for discordance commonly requires review of the original frozen section slide(s) and comparison with permanent sections prepared from residual frozen tissue (ANP.12075). Reasons for discordance and their reported relative frequencies include[4-7]:

- Misinterpretation   25% to 40%
- Specimen (tissue) sampling   30% to 45%
- Block sampling   30% to 38%
- Technical (sectioning) inadequacy   6% to 13%
- Inadequate clinical data   6% to 8%
- Labeling errors   0.5% to 3%

The medical consequence of each discordance should be determined (outcome review) and assigned to an appropriate quality assurance category according to clinical impact:

- No clinical significance
- Minor or questionable clinical significance
- Major or potentially major clinical significance

A Q-Probes study of intraoperative consultations found that two-thirds of consultations were requested to establish/confirm a diagnosis or to confirm adequacy of margins.[8] Regardless of the reasons for the request, the surgical procedure was changed in 39% of cases based upon the intraoperative consultation (intraoperative consultation alone, intraoperative consultation with frozen section diagnosis, or intraoperative consultation with deferred frozen section diagnosis).

Institutions should monitor frozen section discordance and deferral rates and determine the rate of false-positive and false-negative diagnoses of malignancy. If there are significant differences from benchmark rates, a study should be initiated to identify reasons. False-positive diagnoses of malignancy often are more likely to have a negative clinical impact (ie, inappropriate therapy) than false-negative diagnoses, and one may choose to establish a lower threshold for such cases.

Data collection and reporting

A number of variables must be considered when collecting and interpreting quality assurance data on frozen section performance, as follows.

- Differences in case mix potentially can account for differences in diagnostic accuracy of frozen section. A high degree of accuracy can be expected for resection margin assessment, identification or verification of unknown tissue, detection of lymph node metastases (excluding sentinel lymph nodes), and determination of tissue adequacy for further diagnostic studies. However, establishing a new diagnosis of an unknown pathologic process has a greater potential for diagnostic discordance (incorrect diagnosis, or correct but imprecise diagnosis) as well as deferred diagnosis.[9]

- Performance data will depend upon whether case discordance (# discordances / # frozen section cases) is calculated, or whether the number of specimens or the number of blocks (# discordances / # of all individual frozen sections) is utilized in the denominator.

- Calculations of discordance can use the broad comparison of benign versus malignant or be based on more specific diagnostic terminology.

- The discordance rate will be higher if deferred diagnoses are subtracted from the denominator.

- Calculation of frozen section discordance rates might exclude such things as:
  - differences in subtypes or grades of malignancy;
  - cases in which there is no gross lesion (eg, mammographic specimens);
  - frozen section done to determine adequacy for other studies (eg, lymph node for flow cytometry studies); and
  - margins oriented en face (ie, Mohs procedure).

- The number of discordant diagnoses may vary depending on specific tissue site or diagnosis.[6,7] Diagnostic discrepancies due to tissue sampling error or block sampling error are relatively more common in breast biopsies and skin lesions, and certain lesions have a documented low rate of frozen section diagnostic accuracy. For example, the overall diagnostic sensitivity of frozen section for thyroid carcinoma ranges from 60% to 70% but varies depending on the type of carcinoma: 94% for classic papillary thyroid carcinoma, 27% for follicular variant of papillary carcinoma, 29% to 55% for follicular carcinoma, and 0% to 26% for encapsulated (or minimally invasive) follicular carcinoma.[10] Inclusion of encapsulated follicular lesions of the thyroid will increase frozen section discordance and/or deferred diagnosis rates.

All of the above are important methodologic points for comparing individual performances with values quoted in the literature as well as for those attempting to reproduce published benchmarks in their own laboratory.

Benchmark data

ADASP recommends an acceptable accuracy threshold of 3% for intraoperative consultation (ie, # of "Disagreement-Major" cases / # of FS cases), and an acceptable threshold of 10% for "Deferred-Inappropriate" cases.[3] The Mayo Clinic, which routinely performs frozen sections for final diagnoses, has reported a frozen section error rate of 2.2% (0.1% significant errors) and deferred diagnoses in 9.0% of cases.[11] The authors of one study of 1000 consecutive frozen section diagnoses found that "unavoidable" factors, such as the focal nature of some lesion or technical imperfections, ie, those not due to misinterpretation, led to erroneous or deferred diagnoses in about 2% of cases.[12]

In other settings, deferred diagnosis rates of 0.2% to 6.1% have been reported.[5,6] The median frozen section discordant diagnosis rate (corrected for deferred diagnoses) was 1.9%, with a range of 1.0% to 3.7% (10th to 90th percentile) and 1.6% to 4.2% for precise diagnoses. False-positive and false-negative rates for the diagnosis of neoplasm have ranged from 0.15% to 0.6% and 0.61% to 2.5% respectively.[7]

A comparison of characteristics and results of the 1989, 1990, and 1994 Q-Probes studies is shown in Table 6-4. The frozen section deferred diagnosis rates ranged from 3.2% to 4.6%. In one of the studies, 1.2% of the deferrals were categorized as inappropriate.[5] The median frozen section discordant diagnosis rates (corrected for deferred diagnoses) ranged from 1.4% to 1.8%. Of the discordant diagnoses, 2.5% to 5.7% had a major effect, and 19.5% to 28.5% had minimal effect on patient care.[5,6] Discordance rates for blocks, specimens, and cases (corrected for deferred diagnoses) are shown in Table 6-5, and diagnostic performance related to false-negative and false-positive diagnoses for neoplasms is shown in Table 6-6.

The aggregate database in the Q-Probes studies may be used to set benchmarks. An institution's performance compared with the aggregate performance value obtained by peer institutions of similar size may be used as a reference for future monitoring and quantitation of improvements in frozen section consultation. Using the Q-Probes benchmark rates, if diagnostic discordance is greater than 2% and/or the deferred diagnosis rate is greater than 5%, the surgical pathologist should initiate a study to identify problem areas.

Diagnostic accuracy: intradepartmental peer review

Background

Discussions of quality in surgical pathology usually concentrate on diagnostic accuracy or "correctness," which is essentially a matter of informed opinion or peer consensus. Regardless of the case selection methods used, peer review consultations will generally fall into either of two categories, prospective or retrospective, and can be internal or interinstitutional.

Intradepartmental peer review can be performed before the pathology report is released (prospective review) or shortly after the report has been released (sometimes called immediate retrospective review). It usually is considered unnecessary to review every case, so review is often targeted to specific types of specimens. Advantages of prospective peer review are simplicity, integration into common consultative practice patterns, and identification of problems before the final report is issued. Among its drawbacks are lack of comprehensiveness, delayed report turnaround time, and difficulty in identifying specific quality issues. Immediate retrospective peer review offers broad scope (all types of specimens can be included), the opportunity to collect several

Table 6-4. Comparison of characteristics and results of Q-Probes studies[6]

Study Characteristics	Q-Probes Studies		
	1989	1990	1994
No. participating institutions	297	461	233
No. with avg. occupied bed size <300	171 (58%)	235 (51%)	229 (98%)
No. surgical pathology cases	933,751	1,693,331	327,884
No. FS diagnoses	79,647	121,668	18,532
No. FS cases	52,464	90,538	13,364
FS consultation case rate	5.6%	5.3%	4.1%
FS deferred diagnosis rate	4.2%	3.2%	4.6%
Median FS discordance diagnosis rate (corrected for deferred diagnoses)	1.7%	1.4%	1.8%
Range of FS discordant diagnosis rate corrected for deferred diagnoses (10th to 90th percentile)	0% - 5%	0% - 4.2%	0% - 7.5%

Table 6-5. Institutional percentile from frozen section studies[7]

Discordant Diagnosis	All-Institution Percentiles		
	10th	50th	90th
For blocks * (%)	3.9	1.4	0.0
For specimens * (%)	4.2	1.4	0.0
For cases* (%)	4.9	1.8	0.0

* Values were not corrected for deferred frozen section diagnoses.

Table 6-6. Diagnostic performance: false-negative and false-positive diagnoses for neoplasms[7]

Type of Discordance	Percentage of All Discordant FS Diagnoses	Percentage of All FS Diagnoses (Corrected for Deferred Diagnoses)		
		Cases	Specimens	Blocks
False-negative	67.8%	1.42	1.14	0.99
False-positive	11.0%	0.23	0.19	0.16

different types of information, and straightforward identification of quality issues. In order to be an effective quality assurance monitor, this review should be a daily ongoing process and should be completed in a timely fashion (eg, within 48 hours of case sign-out).

Peer review may also take the form of a daily slide conference, or a request for review may be initiated by a clinician because of ambiguity of the diagnosis or a lack of correlation with clinical findings. These requests should be channeled through the pathologist of record, and the results should be included in the department's quality improvement results.

Peer review programs may also encompass other activities, such as:

- Institutional teaching conferences and tumor boards
- Periodic audit of individual pathologist performance
- Random sampling of cases (eg, 25 cases or 1% accessions per month[3])
- Focused audit of departmental files based on topic (eg, endometrial hyperplasia) or case type (eg, prostate resections)
- Audit of cases sent to outside institutions for routine review

Responsibility for each case remains with the original sign-out pathologist. If clinically important diagnostic disagreements occur or a peer consensus cannot be reached, obtaining an expert consultation may be advisable, particularly if there are potential clinical implications. The results of both prospective and retrospective review should be documented, and it has been recommended that the report include a comment that the case has been reviewed when done so prospectively.[3] Any change in diagnosis that has possible patient care implications should elicit a revised or amended report (see also chapter 3).

To achieve the goals of improving diagnostic results and minimizing clinically significant errors, cases selected for review should include those that have the potential for being the most clinically significant, as well as randomly selected cases. Targeted reviews may include all new cancer diagnoses,[13] certain specimen types that are known to have difficult lesions or frequent cancer mimics (eg, prostate and breast), and diagnostic biopsies in "high-risk" settings because of an increased potential for adverse outcome. Second opinion review is best used on clinically important cases and cases that are problem prone as defined by the individual, the group, the clinician, or the literature. Case types associated with increased frequency of malpractice claims include lymphoma, melanoma, and prostate needle biopsies.[14]

While targeted review can provide data on false-positive diagnoses, case selection should also include a method of identifying false-negative diagnoses. This generally requires review of randomly selected cases to identify unexpected errors.

In selecting cases for internal peer review and determining appropriate benchmarks, the following principles should be kept in mind.[13,15]

- Practices that rely on review of abnormal cases alone will not be able to evaluate false-negative errors.

- Review of every case is enormously burdensome and usually not affordable.

- Reviewing only randomly selected cases focuses a disproportionate amount of effort on cases that have a low likelihood of error. Review of such cases may also have a very low level of vigilance.

- Codified strategies for second opinions should be used based on result criticality, existing medical knowledge, statutory regulations, individual departmental experience, individual pathologist experience, and clinical information.

- In addition to highly critical or significant cases and problem-prone cases, second opinion should be considered for rare disorders that have clinical importance as well as new procedures and specimen types.

Among 74 institutions participating in a Q-Probes study of patient safety in anatomic pathology, a variety of prospective and retrospective review processes were used in the quality assurance program[16]:

- Intradepartmental conference for difficult cases (70%)
- Review percentage of cases after sign-out (42%)
- Review all malignancies before sign-out (30%)
- Review percentage of cases before sign-out (26%)
- Review all malignancies after sign-out (8%)
- Review all cases before sign-out (1%)

Data collection and reporting

The prevalence of diagnostic errors is related to many factors[13]:

- Case selection, as described above
- Accuracy of gross specimen examination and adequacy of tissue sampling
- Quality of specimen preparations used for diagnosis
- Availability of special studies used for diagnostic aides
- Adequacy of the classification systems used for diagnostic and prognostic stratification
- Skill of the diagnostician
- Clinical information

For each nonconcurrence resulting from the peer review process, the disagreement and clinical impact (none, minor or possible, major or definite) should be recorded. Disagreement along continuous categories (eg, grading of cervical dysplasia) is associated less often with altered final diagnoses than discrete disagreements due to misinterpretation or oversight.

Diagnostic accuracy and agreement are not necessarily equated, particularly if the review process is not blinded with respect to the initial diagnosis. In addition, disagreements should not be equated with errors. Disagreements, or discrepancies, refer to any difference between the original interpretation and the interpretation after second review.

Renshaw et al[17] have used the following classification.

- **Threshold disagreement:** reflects a difference of opinion, where there is concurrence on the nature of the lesion but not its degree, eg, actinic keratosis versus squamous cell carcinoma in situ or atypical intraductal hyperplasia versus ductal carcinoma in situ
- **Type/grade disagreement:** relates to process type, eg, basal cell versus squamous cell carcinoma, or histologic grade
- **False-negative rate:** relates to screening and measures whether the lesion is recognized
- **False-positive rate:** relates to diagnoses in which the lesion was not present

If upon re-review, the consensus disagreement was important enough to result in a change in the diagnostic report, the original interpretation was regarded as a diagnostic error. Potentially clinically significant errors were those in which treatment or prognosis might be different.

An alternative approach to classifying discrepancies was used by Raab et al in a recent Q-Probes study[16]:

- Change in margin status
- Change in categorical interpretation, eg, benign to malignant

- Change within same category of interpretation, eg, malignant diagnosis changed to different type of malignancy
- Change in patient information
- Typographical error

In this study, the taxonomy of the effect of a pathology discrepancy on patient outcome was based on medical patient-safety literature:

- Harm (significant event): mild, moderate, or severe
- Near miss: discrepancy detected before harm occurred
- No harm (eg, typographical error)

Although the original and second-opinion diagnoses may be in agreement, clinically significant discrepancies may occur in cancer cases because of a report lacking complete or accurate information: gross tumor size, site or extent of involvement, depth of invasion, histologic cell type/grade, regional lymph node status, and surgical margins. The routine use of standardized synoptic reports for cancer resection specimens will minimize errors of omission.

A Q-Probes study[2] examined the frequency and nature of problems caused by inadequate clinical data provided on surgical pathology requisition forms. A 0.73% aggregate rate of cases required additional clinical information for diagnosis (10th to 90th percentile, 3.01% to 0.08%). In 6.1% of cases, there was a substantial change in the diagnosis, requiring a revised report.

Amended report rates, although a useful quality assurance monitor, do not measure error rates, because surveillance and better detection will increase the amended report rate in the absence of a true increase in errors. A Q-Probes study[18] showed that the aggregate median rate of amended reports (all types) was 1.5 per 1000 cases (approximately 0.15%). Of the amended reports, 38.7% were issued to revise the originally issued final diagnoses and 26.5% to revise other reported diagnostic information that was clinically significant. Error detection was most commonly (20.5%) precipitated by a request from a clinician to review the case. The median amended report rates (all types) were stratified by peer slide review mechanism: retrospective, 1.6 per 1000; none, 1.4 per 1000; prospective, 1.2 per 1000; prospective review of a set percentage of cases, 0.94 per 1000. It was suggested that the 90th percentile amended report rate of approximately 0.025% might approximate a "best practices" benchmark.[19]

A high amended report rate should lead to further analysis of the types and sources of errors that contribute to the finding, with a focus on those errors likely to alter patient management, ie, the goal is to reduce clinically significant errors, not amended reports. When monitoring amended report rates, one should not count those issued following preliminary or provisional reports, as those are not amended because of error.

Benchmark data

"Gold standards" for determining what are acceptable and unacceptable individual errors and overall error rates are not well defined. Interinstitutional review and/or clinical follow-up may prove the initial diagnosis correct; even accepted expert opinion for carcinoma is not 100% specific when follow-up material is used as the gold standard.[15] Therefore, a quality assurance program to measure accuracy of diagnoses should have a built-in mechanism of outcome review based upon correlation of biopsy diagnosis with resection specimen.

The sensitivity of the review process is critical for establishing benchmarks.[15,20] Blinded retrospective review (ie, without knowledge of the original diagnosis or history) can be an effective

Table 6-7. Summary of error rates in surgical pathology*

Reference	No. of Cases Reviewed	Type of Review	Case Selection	(Total) Error Rate (%)	Significant Error Rate (%)
Safrin and Bark[22]	5,397	Prospective	Consecutive	0.5	0.26
Whitehead et al[23]	3,000	Prospective	Consecutive	7.8	0.96
Lind et al[24]	2,694	Prospective	Diagnostic bx's	13.0	1.2
Lind et al[24]	480	Retrospective	Random	12.0	1.7

* Modified from Renshaw[15]

Table 6-8. Number (%) of surgical pathology errors according to type*

Reference	Case Selection	Error Type						
		False Neg.	False Pos.	Threshold	Type & Grade	Missed Margin	Other	Total
Safrin and Bark[22]	Consecutive	6 (43)	2 (14)	2 (14)	2 (14)	0 (0)	2 (14)	14
Whitehead et al[23]	Consecutive	9 (14)	8 (13)	7 (11)	12 (19)	1 (<1)	26 (41)	63
Lind et al[24]	Diagnostic biopsies	21 (40)	3 (1)	9 (17)	4 (8)	5 (10)	10 (19)	52

* Modified from Renshaw[15]

method for quality improvement in surgical pathology. In the study by Renshaw and colleagues,[21] complete agreement was found in 567 of 592 cases (96%). Threshold disagreements were most common. Blinded review missed 7 cases (1.2%). The review process had a sensitivity for both abnormality and for malignancy of 98%, and the specificity of the technique was 100% (ie, no false-positives). In a more recent study, which reported the results of blinded review of 5000 sequential biopsy cases that were heavily weighted to dermatopathology cases, complete agreement occurred in approximately 91% of cases.[17] Again, diagnostic disagreement was primarily due to threshold differences: 292 of 444 cases. The technique had a sensitivity of greater than 99% (19 false-negative cases). Blinded review has the additional advantage of identifying clinically significant false-negative cases.

Available data suggest that the greatest source of error is with false-negative diagnoses. In two of three studies of consecutive cases or biopsy specimens, false-negative diagnoses, ie, completely missing the lesion, comprised approximately 40% of errors (Tables 6-7 and 6-8). Total error rates ranged from 0.5% to 13%, and significant error rates ranged from 0.26% to 1.7%. With the blinded review process, Renshaw et al[17] found that diagnostic disagreement led to a change in the original report (true error) in 0.1% of cases, and the clinically significant error rate was 0.08%.

The study by Lind and colleagues[24] demonstrated minimal difference in major error and minor error (clinically insignificant) detection rate between prospective review of consecutive cases and retrospective review of randomly selected cases: 1.2% and 12.9% versus 1.7% and 11.5%. Another study has shown that retrospective review of 2% of cases detected important errors in 1.2% of reports.[25] Renshaw et al[26] reported findings of in-house consultation (ie, prospective review) of 20%

of all surgical pathology cases, and disagreements occurred in 2% of their case volume. Of the cases reviewed, initial complete agreement was found in 89.5%. Using the final sign-out as the "gold standard," 1.1% of cases were classified as false-negative, 0.3% as false-positive, 0.9% as differences in type, and 8.2% as differences in threshold. Disagreements were thought to be potentially clinically significant in 2.8% of cases.

Based upon these limited number of studies, it would appear that a reasonable threshold for clinically significant errors detected by surgical pathology case review would be less than 2%. Establishing an overall threshold for discrepancies (major and minor) is more problematic. In the study by Whitehead and colleagues,[23] the final diagnosis was modified in 2.2% of cases, which might suggest a reasonable overall threshold for major and minor disagreements of less than 3%. It has been suggested that because published error rates are low, a relatively large number of cases need to be reviewed and a relatively great difference in error rate needs to exist in order to show a significant difference in performance in surgical pathology.[27]

A recent Q-Probes study[16] established a mean multi-institutional discrepancy frequency for surgical pathology cases (related to secondary review) of 6.8%. Although the majority of discrepancies had no effect on patient care, 5.3% had a moderate or marked effect, and 1.1% of anatomic pathology (surgical and cytology) cases reviewed were associated with a harmful significant event. Some of the secondary review methods detected more error than other methods. For example, clinician-directed review detected a discrepancy (23% of cases) more frequently than random review (4.3%). Error frequency based on extradepartmental conference review was 7.1%. Additionally, the reason for case review correlated with patient outcome in discrepant cases. "Harm" occurred more frequently in discrepant cases that were reviewed at the request of the clinician (23.5%) and interdepartmental conference (25%). These data indicate that benchmarking and establishing meaningful thresholds requires correlation of error frequencies with particular review practices and existing laboratory error reduction programs.

Wakely et al[28] developed an alternative method of evaluating diagnostic performance that compares diagnostic patterns of individual surgical pathologists. By establishing a standardized ratio (observed to expected rate of diagnosis) with a 95% confidence interval, they were able to determine rates of relative overdiagnosis and underdiagnosis for common types of biopsies that had limited numbers of bottom-line diagnoses (eg, TURPs, bladder biopsies, endometrial curettings). This method identifies inconsistencies in diagnosis rates, ie, aberrant rates, rather than diagnostic inaccuracies, and provides pathologists with a profile of diagnostic patterns in comparison with their peers.

Renshaw has suggested that in order to be comparable, error rates in surgical pathology must be reported in reference to disease incidence and not to overall caseload.[15] Until appropriate surrogates are developed, including examining only diagnostic biopsies, data will be difficult to interpret and misleading with respect to accurately measuring the overall error rates, which are currently underestimated. Examples of surrogate monitors, comparable to monitoring ASCUS/SIL ratios in Pap smears, include the ratio of atypical ductal hyperplasia of the breast to the number of image-guided core biopsies performed for calcifications[29] or high-grade PIN/cancer ratios in prostate needle biopsy specimens.

Diagnostic accuracy: interinstitutional peer review

Background

Interinstitutional (external) case review provides an additional mechanism for evaluating diagnostic accuracy at the original institution. It is a form of retrospective peer review and should be distinguished from formal extradepartmental consultations that are requested because of diagnostic uncertainty or lack of peer group consensus. A Q-Probes study[30] evaluating surgical pathology consultation practices has shown an aggregate consultation rate of 0.5% (median 0.7%). Another study[31] showed a higher consultation rate for a community hospital than a tertiary care medical center (4.6% versus 0.3%).

External review is generally initiated for one of the following reasons:

- Patient request for second opinion
- Clinician request for second opinion
- Pathologist request for confirmation of a diagnosis
- Institutional request because of patient transfer and need for diagnostic review by a pathologist at the new treating institution

Recommendations for extradepartmental consultation have been developed by ADASP,[32] and a consensus conference focused on second opinions in diagnostic anatomic pathology as a mechanism for error reduction.[13] It is recommended that treating institutions establish a policy of mandatory second opinion on nonemergent cases for which major therapeutic interventions are planned based on a tissue (or cytologic) diagnosis. Diagnostic discrepancies with the referring institution should be resolved before definitive therapy. A recent survey showed that only 50% of responding hospitals required in-house review, and approximately 87% either encouraged or required this review.[33] In comparing types of practice, 76% of academic-tertiary care centers and only 33% of community general hospitals had this requirement.

When evaluating published data for error detection rates revealed by interinstitutional review and attempting to establish a reasonable benchmark for performance, the following factors need to be taken into account.

- Interinstitutional review is not an effective method of detecting the greatest source of errors: false-negative diagnoses.

- Cases sent as true consults ordinarily are not included in the calculated percentage of disagreements, though monitoring the level of agreement with these types of cases may be useful in evaluating the value of external consultation.

- The risk for discordance on external review varies with different organ systems.

- As with internal peer review, thresholds for overall diagnostic discordance rates and significant error rates should be distinguished.

- Comparison of data is difficult because of varying definitions of "significant diagnostic differences" or "major disagreements." In general, these should refer to discordant diagnoses that result in a major modification in therapy, change in evaluation, or alteration in prognosis. Reasons for discordant interpretation with clinical impact in oncological pathology review include false-positives, false-negatives, change in tumor type/grade, resection margin status, stage change, and threshold.

Table 6-9. Interinstitutional review: summary of error rates detected by mandatory second opinion

Reference	Total Error Rate (%)	Significant Error Rate (%)
Kronz et al[36]	Not known	1.4%
Abt et al[37]	9.1% *	5.8%
Gupta et al[33]	1% - 30%	2% - 5% (avg.)
Malhotra et al[35]	11.6%	Not known
Weir et al[34]	6.8%	3.7%

* 7.8% error rate for surgical pathology specimens;
   21% error rate for cytopathology and fine-needle aspiration biopsy specimens.

Table 6-10. Interinstitutional review: summary of error rates by organ systems

Organ System	Reference	Total Error Rate (%)	Significant Error Rate (%)
Lymphoma	40	Hodgkin 16.7% Non-Hodgkin 27.3%	Not known
Neuropathology	41	43%	8.8% (incl. consult cases)
	42	Not known	8.6%
	43	23%	3.7%
Gynecology-Oncology	44	Not known	2.0%
Oncology	45	16.9%	4.7%
EMB/EMC*	39	Not known	24%
Ovarian Ca	46	12.7%	4.4% false-positive
Sarcoma	47	Not known	22% false-positive
Prostate (NB)	48	Not known	1.3% false-positive

* Endometrial biopsy/endometrial curettings

- Discrepant pathology review can result from additional sectioning (re-cuts should be reviewed by sign-out pathologist before sending case out) or additional testing. In one report,[34] performing or repeating immunohistochemistry on cases referred for treatment or second opinion resulted in a clinically significant change in diagnosis in 20% of cases. Of these cases, 47% had prior immunohistochemistry, which was repeated or added to. The application of molecular diagnostic techniques will likely affect error detection as well.

Data collection and reporting

Data collection and reporting may be performed in a fashion similar to that described for intradepartmental peer review.

Benchmark data

Overall diagnostic discrepancy rates in surgical pathology detected by mandatory second opinion on referral cases have ranged from 1% to 30% (Table 6-9). Significant error rates have generally ranged from 1.4% to 5.8%, including surgical pathology and cytopathology/fine-needle aspiration biopsy specimens. In the report by Malhotra et al,[35] interinstitutional review disclosed 10% cancer-related discrepancies requiring a change in clinical evaluation or therapy.

Table 6-10 shows diagnostic discordance rates according to organ system.[39-48] The largest error rates are reported for lymphomas, neuropathology cases (majority typing/grading), and GYN-tract specimens (especially endometrial curettings/biopsies). Significant errors were detected in 1.3% to 24% of cases. In 4.6% to 13.5% of cases, follow-up supported the original diagnosis over the second opinion.[36-38]

Based upon published reports, a reasonable threshold for overall discrepancy rates between original and outside review diagnosis is 10%. ADASP estimates that an acceptable threshold for clinically significant disagreement following arbitration is 2%, as applied to those cases in which it is decided that the correct interpretation is that from the outside institution.[3]

Postanalytic variables: report adequacy and integrity

Patrick L. Fitzgibbons, MD

Report adequacy

Background

Measures to assess the adequacy of pathology reporting are an important component of a department's quality improvement plan and serve as one indicator of quality of care. Ensuring the adequacy of pathology reporting also improves the value of disease surveillance systems. While this monitor encompasses both report accuracy and report completeness, the latter is generally easier for laboratories to measure.

Adequacy of pathology reporting is probably most easily monitored for cancer cases, and most published benchmarks on report adequacy relate to cancer reporting. In tumor cases, the report must include all information necessary for patient care (see LAP checklist item ANP.12350). Many studies have shown that standardized reporting forms, including synoptic reports or checklists, are highly effective in improving report adequacy, particularly for cancer reporting.[49-52] Several recent reports confirm the value of checklists in reducing the frequency of missing data elements in cancer cases.[53,54]

For those institutions with cancer programs that are accredited by the American College of Surgeons Commission on Cancer (CoC), special monitoring of report adequacy is required. The CoC Cancer Program Standard 4.6 mandates that 90% of pathology reports that include a cancer diagnosis contain all the scientifically validated data elements outlined in the surgical case summary checklists of the CAP's publication, *Reporting on Cancer Specimens.*[55] The required, scientifically validated data elements are the nonasterisked elements in the checklists. The CoC does not require the actual use of the checklists, and the order and format in which these data elements are reported is at the discretion of the pathologist.

Studies of quality improvement in surgical pathology often focus on diagnostic accuracy, but increasing numbers of studies of report completeness are now available. In a retrospective analysis of randomly selected surgical pathology reports, Ramsay and Gallagher found omissions of pathology

Table 6-11. Monitors used to gauge report adequacy

	Data Element
Specimens of any type	Patient identifiers
	Pertinent clinical history
	Specimen site
	Statement of specimen adequacy (when appropriate)
	Adequate macroscopic description
	Clear diagnostic terminology
	Transcription accuracy
Primary cancer specimens	Tumor size
	Histologic type
	Histologic grade (if appropriate)
	Extent or depth of invasion (if appropriate)
	Number of lymph nodes examined
	Number of nodes with metastases (if any)
	Status of surgical margins (if appropriate)
Image-guided biopsies	A comment on specimen adequacy
	A comment on whether the biopsy findings correlate with the imaging findings (eg, whether the findings explain the targeted abnormality)
	The presence of calcifications in a biopsy performed for that reason

reporting that affected patient management.[25] In assessing accuracy and clarity of the gross description and microscopic diagnosis, they found "satisfactory" reports in an average of 89% of cases. Perhaps more importantly, these authors showed that reporting problems that affect patient management can be identified by systematic review of pathology reports.

Monitoring for report completeness may be particularly useful in identifying problems with more recently adopted pathology parameters. For example, two studies of pathology reports of rectal carcinomas[56,57] showed high rates of reporting of traditional pathologic parameters such as tumor type, tumor size, histologic grade and extent of invasion, but a significantly lower rate for radial margin assessment (48% and 63%, respectively).

Data collection and reporting

While a department should have a regular method of monitoring report adequacy, most often by periodic review of completed surgical pathology reports, one can choose to monitor different specimen types, cancer types, or specific data elements for a given time period.[58] Examples of the kinds of monitors one may choose to follow are listed in Table 6-11.

For CoC-approved cancer programs, the institution's cancer committee must monitor and report compliance with the requirement to include all scientifically validated data elements. At a minimum, the committee must review pathology reports for a random sample of 10% of the annual analytic cases, or a maximum of 300 cases each year, to document compliance with this standard. The CoC has developed a template to assist in this monitoring (Figure 6-1).

Figure 6-1. American College of Surgeons Commission on Cancer compliance monitoring template

CoC Quality Control of Pathology Reports Tool

This tool is provided to document compliance with Standard 4.6.

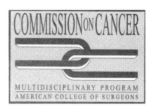

Figures are based on the cancer committee quality review of cancer registry abstracts. A minimum of 10 percent of analytic caseload must be reviewed annually (to a maximum of 300 cases).

Month/Time Period of Audit: Primary Sites Chosen to Audit:

Number of cases abstracted this period: Number of cases audited this period:

Criteria:
1. Pathology report includes cancer-related diagnosis.
2. Scientifically validated data elements are completed.
3. Other criteria established by the cancer committee.

Patient ID	1	2	3	Comments

Criteria

Directions:
1. If the criterion is met, put an (X) in the appropriate box.
2. If the criterion is not met, put a zero (0) in the appropriate box.
3. If the criterion does not apply, put (NA) in the appropriate box.
4. Comment on all zero (0) responses.
5. Identify the follow-up action required, if any.

Results of Review:

____ Percentage of cases with pathology reports including cancer diagnosis.

____ Percentage of pathology reports that include scientifically validated data elements.

Identified errors and proposed resolution:

Signature of auditor (physician): _____ Date: _____

Date presented to cancer committee: _____

Source: American College of Surgeons Commission on Cancer. Reproduced with permission.

Table 6-12. Rectal cancer reports[57]

	Frequency*
Tumor type	100%
Depth of invasion	100%
Histologic grade	99%
Distance to nearest margin	98%
Number of nodes examined	93%
Status of radial margin	63%
Location of positive nodes	42%

* Percentage of pathology reports with information present

Benchmark data

Several studies have addressed the issue of report adequacy and provide useful data on specific cancer sites (see Tables 6-12 through 6-15). These studies monitored the frequency with which specific data elements were included in pathology reports, but it should be noted that some were done before widespread adoption of synoptic reporting, which as stated previously has been shown to improve completeness of reporting. Thus, these percentages may not necessarily represent appropriate benchmarks applicable to current practice.

Report integrity

Background

Monitoring the accuracy and completeness of pathology reporting also requires ensuring the integrity of reports that are electronically reproduced.[62] Reports that are accessed by computers outside the pathology department or that are transmitted by electronic devices (eg, autofax, off-site printer) constitute part of the medical record and may be the only report seen by health care workers at distant locations. A study of electronic laboratory reporting showed that automatic reporting was substantially more rapid than paper-based reporting, and that errors were most often related to the use of free text.[63]

Table 6-13. Breast cancer reports[59]

	Frequency*
Invasive carcinoma	
Tumor size	94%
Tumor type	99.6%
Status of margins	87%
Histologic grade	84%
Presence or absence of DCIS	79%
Presence or absence of vascular invasion	61%
Ductal carcinoma in situ	
Extent or size of DCIS	49%
Presence or absence of necrosis	41%
Grade of DCIS	39%

* Percentage of pathology reports with information present

Table 6-14. Lung cancer reports[60]

	Frequency*
Tumor size	97%
Tumor type	99%
Presence or absence of tumor at bronchial margin	91%
Histologic grade	89%
Presence or absence of lymphatic invasion	24%
Presence or absence of venous invasion	23%
Presence or absence of visceral pleural invasion	67%
Status of lymph nodes	96%

* Percentage of pathology reports with information present

Table 6-15. Urinary bladder cancer reports[61]

	Frequency*
Invasive or noninvasive specified in report	92%
Histologic type of invasive cancer stated	99%
Histologic grade of invasive cancer stated	97%
Histologic grade of noninvasive cancer stated	98%
Depth of invasion stated in report (for invasive cancers)	53%
Absence of invasion stated in report (for noninvasive cancers)	94%

* Percentage of pathology reports with information present

Electronic reports must be periodically reviewed and compared with the original pathology report to detect errors in data transmission, storage, or processing (GEN.43500). In addition to periodically reviewing and approving the content and format of computer generated reports, video displays of reports should be reviewed to verify that patient results are accurately transmitted and that all patient test results are available and effectively communicated. Attention also should be paid to comments, addendum reports, and other special situations to ensure that all essential information in the original report is clearly and completely communicated.

Data collection and benchmark data

There have been no systematic studies of the final step in surgical pathology reporting—receipt by the responsible clinician with appropriate action taken—but clinical laboratory studies of this phase of the test cycle suggest that this is an area with a high potential for quality improvement. One Q-Probes study of elevated calcium levels found that clinicians were frequently unaware of abnormal results when they were not expecting an abnormality.[64] While there are no published benchmarks available for report receipt, a department may devise methods to periodically monitor this phase, for example by periodically surveying the clinicians or their office staffs about this phase of the test cycle.

Turnaround time

Cheryl M. Coffin, MD

Introduction

Turnaround times (TAT) for surgical pathology frozen sections, biopsies, and large specimens are key indicators of the overall function of the service and are a critical component of quality practice because of their impact on clinical management of patients. In today's medical environment, the timeliness of communication is as important as diagnostic accuracy and report completeness. Results of turnaround-time studies can be used to modify structures, processes, and systems, which can contribute to better patient outcome. The elements that affect turnaround time involve complex aspects of the hospital and anatomic pathology laboratory, with many technical, clerical, and human interpretive processes.[65-67] The importance of turnaround time is reflected in the CAP LAP Anatomic Pathology Checklist requirements for both frozen sections and surgical pathology.

Different types of specimens vary in their impact on clinical care through the immediacy of decisions or actions based on the diagnostic results. Publications from ADASP[3] and from the CAP Q-Probes studies[66-70] advocate separating turnaround time assessments for frozen sections, small diagnostic biopsies, and large or complex specimens. Further recommendations have been published that turnaround time data collection be performed continuously and stratified by individual pathologists in order to assess technical and clerical processes and the comparative efficiency of pathologists.[65,66,71] Turnaround time data can be used to incrementally enhance surgical pathology processes through definition of goals, collection and analysis of data, and process modification and reevaluation.[72,73] Finally, turnaround time information may be used for peer review and performance based hospital credentialing of individual pathologists.[65,66]

Frozen sections

Background

Frozen section turnaround time has a critical impact on operative management. Data from CAP Q-Probes suggest that 90% of frozen section block turnaround times can be completed within 20 minutes, measured from the time that the pathologist receives a frozen section specimen to the time that a diagnosis is reported to the surgeon.[69] The LAP addresses this through ANP.11820, which requires that the laboratory periodically evaluate turnaround time for intraoperative frozen sections, documenting the reason(s) if 90% are not completed within 20 minutes.

Data collection and reporting

Frozen section turnaround time data can be collected easily if the time of receipt of the specimen and the time of reporting are recorded. This can be done by computer or on written frozen section report forms for all frozen section cases, and can be included in the final report in the section documenting frozen section results. Monitoring of frozen section turnaround time may be done monthly as part of the routine anatomic pathology quality assurance plan, or on a less frequent basis if there has been documentation of previous performance within thresholds. The suggested benchmark based on Q-Probes data is that 90% of frozen section block turnaround times are completed within 20 minutes.[69] Complicated cases with multiple simultaneous frozen sections may be excluded from this benchmark. Outliers can be explained in summary fashion in a regular frozen section turnaround time quality assurance report. An example is shown in Figure 6-2.

Benchmark data

The suggested benchmark based on Q-Probes data is that 90% of frozen section block turnaround times are completed within 20 minutes.[69] Q-Probes data from 32,868 frozen sections performed in 700 institutions revealed that turnaround times exceeding 20 minutes occurred more often when more than one pathologist or when residents and medical students participated in the frozen section procedure, when pathologists had to retrieve and review previous case material during the frozen section procedure, when multiple simultaneous frozen section specimens were received, when a final frozen section diagnosis could not be reached, and when technical problems occurred.[69] Shorter turnaround times were associated with scheduled frozen sections and smaller hospital size. The effects on turnaround time of new frozen section techniques, such as rapid special stains and immunohistochemistry, and new medical procedures, such as sentinel lymph node biopsy, have yet to be determined.[73,74] There are limited data about frozen section turnaround time in teaching hospitals.[75]

Preanalytic variables, such as delivery time from the operating room to the laboratory, which influence frozen section turnaround time, have not been assessed because they are generally considered outside of the control of the laboratory and the pathologists. Other preanalytic factors influencing turnaround time include the site of origin of the specimen, the diagnostic purpose of the procedure, and the need to defer the diagnosis because of complex diagnostic criteria, as in classification of certain types of neoplasms. Elements within the control of pathologists include the number and type of people participating in the procedure, review of previous case material, juggling of simultaneous frozen section requests, and anticipation and prospective prevention of instrument malfunctions. Generally complicated cases with multiple frozen sections, such as skin for evaluation

Figure 6-2. Frozen section turnaround time report

Time period reviewed: _____

Total frozen section blocks: _____

Number exceeding 20-minute threshold: _____

% exceeding threshold: _____

Data Summary for Cases Exceeding 20 Minutes

Accession Number	Diagnosis	TAT	Pathologists	Comment

Conclusion/recommendation:

Action taken:

Follow-up required:

Figure 6-3. Surgical pathology turnaround time report

Time period reviewed: _____

Total surgical pathology cases: _____

Number exceeding threshold: _____

% exceeding threshold: _____

Data Summary for Cases Exceeding Threshold

Accession Number	Diagnosis	TAT	Pathologists	Comment

Conclusion/recommendation:

Action taken:

Follow-up required:

of multiple margins, are not expected to meet the 20-minute CAP LAP benchmark. A survey of quality assurance practices in pediatric pathology departments revealed that 7 of 29 institutions surveyed monitored frozen section turnaround time.[76]

Surgical pathology specimens

Background

Surgical pathology turnaround times have been the topic of publications from ADASP,[3] Q-Probes,[66-70] a survey of pediatric pathology departments,[76] and individual communications from institutions inside and outside the United States.[65,71,72,77-80] ADASP has recommended separate analysis of turnaround time for different types of specimens (Table 6-16), including retrospective monitoring through random case review, and considers an acceptable threshold for these turnaround times to be 80%. The CAP has addressed surgical pathology turnaround time through the LAP AP Checklist item ANP.12150, which asks: Are reports on routine cases completed within 2 working days? The AP Checklist notes that unusual, complex, or special specimens may require prolonged fixation, additional times for special stains, and greater reporting time, but points out that the question is primarily concerned with the majority of routine specimens.

Data collection and reporting

Surgical pathology turnaround times are calculated by subtracting the accession date from the verification date, excluding weekends, holidays, or other times when pathologists and technical support are not available. This information may be calculated electronically, or the data may be collected manually. The pathologist responsible for quality assurance or the director of anatomic pathology has the discretion to decide the frequency of turnaround time monitoring and whether to separate biopsies, routine large specimens, and complex large specimens requiring special studies. The simplest approach is to measure the percentage of reports completed within the 2-day threshold contained in the LAP AP Checklist. According to Q-Probes data, this goal was met for 95% of routine biopsies and 91% of routine complex specimens.[65,66] Depending on the size of the laboratory and initial findings of turnaround time studies, continuous assessment may be performed, or periodic sampling with assessment of turnaround time may be done. An example of a report which can be adapted for review of biopsies, routine large specimens, complex specimens, or individual pathologist turnaround times is shown in Figure 6-3.

Table 6-16. ADASP benchmarks and thresholds for surgical pathology turnaround times[3]

Type of Specimen	Report Finalization	Threshold
Rush biopsies	2 days	80%
Biopsies	3 days	80%
Surgical specimens	3 days	80%
Additional Time for Special Procedures		
Overnight fixation	1 day	
Decalcification	1 day	
Resubmission	1-2 days	
Recuts	1 day	
Immunohistochemistry	1-2 days	
Electron microscopy	2-3 days	
Intradepartmental consultation	1 day	

Table 6-17. CAP LAP guidelines and Q-Probes results for surgical pathology[66-70]

Type of Specimen	Turnaround Time	Threshold
Frozen sections	20 minutes	90%
Routine biopsies	2 days	95%
Routine complex specimens	2 days	91%

Benchmark data

The benchmarks and thresholds are summarized in Tables 6-16 and 6-17. A Q-Probes study of biopsies and complex specimens from surgical pathology laboratories concluded that a 2-day turnaround time is a reasonable goal and was met in 95% of routine biopsies and 91% of routine complex surgical specimens.[66] Among 15,725 biopsy cases from 525 laboratories, 79% overall were completed within 1 working day, 95% within 2 working days, and 98% within 3 working days. In 90% of laboratories, all biopsy reports were completed by the second working day, and in 95%, by the third working day. The mean turnaround time for biopsies was 1.2 days. Longer biopsy turnaround times were associated with a larger institutional size, greater number of surgical pathologists, the volume of cases processed, technical procedures resulting in delayed slides, integration of resident training with biopsy sign-out, and decreased staffing levels of histotechnicians, histotechnologists, and transcriptionists. Among 4298 complex specimens from 489 laboratories, 68% required routine processing and 32% required special handling. Overall, 56% of complex specimens were completed within 1 working day, 81% within 2 working days, 91% within 3 working days, and 95% by 4 working days. The mean turnaround time for complex specimens was 1.5 days overall, with 1.3 days for routine specimens and 2.6 days for specimens that required special handling. Longer turnaround time was associated with hospital size of greater than 450 beds, specimen grossing responsibilities by residents only, availability of slides after 12 PM, resident involvement in case sign-out, interposition of a day between the availability of slides and the final sign-out, and a greater number of surgical pathologists. Special procedures contributed an average of 1.3 additional days to turnaround time.

A separate Q-Probes study examined biopsies performed in small hospitals, generally less than 200 beds.[70] In a study of 5384 surgical biopsies in 157 small hospitals, 85.9% were completed within 2 days, and 88.3% were completed within 4 days. Factors influencing a shorter turnaround time included a yearly surgical case load of greater than 2000 cases per full-time equivalent pathologist, availability of pathology support services on site, and hospital and laboratory accreditation by the Joint Commission on Accreditation of Healthcare Organizations and the CAP.

Published information about turnaround time from other institutions, organizations, and countries is limited. Anatomic pathology turnaround times in academic medical centers were documented to average 3.15 days for both biopsies and larger specimens in a study from the Medical University of South Carolina.[71] This was attributed to a combination of resident involvement in sign-out, performance of special stains, need for intradepartmental and extradepartmental consultations, need to obtain additional clinical information, and performance of molecular studies prior to final diagnosis. A survey of pediatric hospitals revealed that less than half routinely measured surgical pathology turnaround times.[76] Longer turnaround time and different benchmarks have been established outside of the United States, with acceptable turnaround times in the range of 2 to 7 days.[72,77-79]

Further considerations

The critical nature of the information contained in frozen section and surgical pathology reports makes acceptable turnaround times important to patients, pathologists, clinicians, and administrators.[71] For patients, treatment and other therapeutic decisions depend on the information contained in the pathology report. For pathologists, turnaround times may be used as managerial tools; for workload, scheduling, and technical and clerical processes; as a justification for technical procedural changes, such as rapid diagnostic tissue preparation; as an indicator for development of remedial measures; as a way to substantiate good service or to manage complaints; and as a way to measure individual and departmental performance and competitive viability. For clinicians, timely pathology reports affect length of stay, ability to complete medical records, and economic factors related to reimbursement. For hospital administrators, turnaround time information provides a measure of the overall efficiency and time limits of a department and possibly its financial competitiveness in a community or region.

Factors affecting surgical pathology turnaround time are complex because of the many steps in the preanalytic, analytic, and postanalytic processes.[65,66,80,81] Specimen procurement, specimen transport, and specimen accessioning, with identification and correction of errors, are all important preanalytic factors that are not under the direct control of the pathologist. Analytic factors include how gross dissection and preparation are performed; whether residents, histotechnologists, and pathologists' assistants are involved in gross dissections; histology laboratory staffing; technology and instrumentation; slide preparation times; pathologist workload and efficiency; diagnostic complexity; and the need for special procedures. Extra time is necessary in the analytic phase for overnight fixation, decalcification, resubmission of tissue, obtaining recuts or blocks, immunohistochemistry, molecular diagnostic tests, electron microscopy, and consultations.[3,65,71]

Postanalytic factors include availability, efficiency, and accuracy of transcription; the need for report editing; methods of report finalization; report transmittal (electronic, mail, fax, courier); time to report charting; and time to report interpretation by physicians caring for the patient. While some aspects of the postanalytic process may be influenced by the pathologists, mail systems, charting, and report interpretation are usually beyond the realm of influence of a pathology department. These considerations cover the entire test cycle period. For the surgical pathology laboratory, selected aspects of the test cycle involving the intralaboratory and intradepartmental processes will yield information that can be used most effectively to improve turnaround time.

Customer satisfaction

Raouf E. Nakhleh, MD

Background

The test cycle in surgical pathology encompasses multiple steps that ultimately lead to the production of diagnostic information, which is disseminated to our customers, primarily physicians, who need this information to manage their patients. Although not frequently discussed in training programs, satisfying physicians' informational needs—or customer satisfaction—is an essential part of surgical pathology. The LAP addresses the question of customer satisfaction in the Laboratory General Checklist (GEN.20367). Customer satisfaction is complex and does not necessarily relate to diagnostic accuracy, timeliness, or cost of service. In many instances, there may be no problem with the diagnosis or turnaround time, but the customer is still unsatisfied.

Overall customer satisfaction involves factors such as communication, appropriateness, and expectations. For example, it may be that the appropriate time frame for processing, producing, and delivering a diagnostic report on a surgical resection specimen is 2 days, and the responsible pathologist renders an appropriate diagnosis within this time frame. However, if the surgeon expects

Figure 6-4. Sample anatomic pathology customer satisfaction survey

Please indicate your level of satisfaction with Anatomic Pathology services

	1 Poor	2 Below Average	3 Average	4 Good	5 Excellent
1. Overall satisfaction rating					
2. Quality of professional interactions					
3. Diagnostic accuracy					
4. Pathologist responsiveness for problems					
5. Pathologist accessibility for frozen sections					
6. Tumor board presentations					
7. Courtesy of secretarial and technical staff					
8. Teaching conferences and courses					
9. Communication of relevant information					
10. Notification of significant abnormal results					
11. Timeliness of reporting					

the report in 1 day, he or she will not be satisfied. Customer satisfaction therefore requires attention to communication and physician education along with delivery of an accurate diagnosis in a timely fashion.

There have been few studies on this topic in anatomic pathology. A recent CAP Q-Probes study addressed overall customer satisfaction in anatomic pathology,[82] and past Q-Probes have assessed various aspects of customer satisfaction. For example, in a study of mammographically-directed breast biopsies, Nakhleh et al also examined physician's expectations compared with final report content.[50] These studies may provide a framework for the development of monitors for overall customer satisfaction.

Data collection and reporting

Data collection may be done in a fashion similar to the Q-Probes study of overall customer satisfaction.[82] In that study, the primary quality indicator was an overall satisfaction score on a scale of 1 to 5, with 1 representing poor and 5 representing excellent. Along with the overall satisfaction score, various aspects of anatomic pathology may be examined, such as the quality of professional interaction, diagnostic accuracy, the pathologist's responsiveness to problems, the pathologist's accessibility for frozen sections, tumor board presentations, courtesy of secretarial and technical staff, communication of relevant information, teaching conferences and courses, notification of significant or abnormal results, and timeliness of report. Each of these measures may also be given a grade of 1 to 5.

Table 6-18. Distribution of institutional overall satisfaction scores

	Percentile		
	10th	50th	90th
Overall satisfaction rating	4.0	4.4	4.7

Table 6-19. Distribution of institutional percentiles with respect to the percentage of excellent/good rating for each service category

	Percentile		
	10th	50th	90th
Quality of professional interactions	81.8	96.3	100
Diagnostic accuracy	82.6	96.1	100
Pathologist responsiveness for problems	82.6	93.6	100
Pathologist accessibility for frozen sections	75.0	93.3	100
Tumor board presentations	75.0	93.1	100
Courtesy of secretarial and technical staff	81.3	93.0	100
Teaching conferences and courses	62.5	88.2	100
Communication of relevant information	69.6	88.5	100
Notification of significant abnormal results	64.7	86.3	100
Timeliness of reporting	56.3	79.8	94.0

Results may be reported as an average of all responding physicians or as the percentage of those with an excellent/good rating versus those with a below average/poor rating. In addition, open-ended questions can be included in the survey to solicit more information regarding laboratory services. Figure 6-4 may be used as a model for collecting this type of data. Some aspects of practice may be deleted from this form and others added, as needed.

If this type of survey has not been performed in the past, a broad initial mailing to all of the laboratory's customers should be considered, with subsequent surveys having a narrower focus depending on perceived problem areas. In general, repetitive survey of a captive set of customers may lose its effectiveness if done too often. It is recommended that this type of survey be conducted annually or biannually.

Benchmark data

In the Q-Probes study of customer satisfaction in anatomic pathology, the overall median satisfaction score was 4.4 (range 1 through 5, where 1=poor and 5=excellent). The percentile ranking is shown in Table 6-18. The percentages of responses with excellent/good ratings for various categories of services are shown in Table 6-19.

References

1. Nakhleh RE, Zarbo RJ. Surgical pathology specimen identification and accessioning: a College of American Pathologists Q-Probes study of 1,004,115 cases from 417 institutions. *Arch Pathol Lab Med.* 1996;120:227-233.

2. Nakhleh RE, Gephardt G, Zarbo RJ. Necessity of clinical information in surgical pathology: a College of American Pathologists Q-Probes study of 771,475 surgical pathology cases from 341 institutions. *Arch Pathol Lab Med.* 1999;123:615-619.

3. Association of Directors of Anatomic and Surgical Pathology. Recommendations on quality control and quality assurance in anatomic pathology. *Am J Surg Pathol.* 1991;15:1007-1009.

4. Howanitz PJ, Hoffman GG, Zarbo RJ. The accuracy of frozen-section diagnoses in 34 hospitals. *Arch Pathol Lab Med.* 1990;114:355-359.

5. Zarbo RJ, Hoffman GG, Howanitz PJ. Interinstitutional comparison of frozen-section consultation: a College of American Pathologist Q-Probes Study of 79,647 consultations in 297 North American institutions. *Arch Pathol Lab Med.* 1991;115:1187-1194.

6. Novis DA, Gephardt GN, Zarbo RJ. Interinstitutional comparison of frozen section consultation in small hospitals: a College of American Pathologists Q-Probes study of 18,532 frozen section consultation diagnoses in 233 small hospitals. *Arch Pathol Lab Med.* 1996;120:1087-1093.

7. Gephardt GN, Zarbo RJ. Interinstitutional comparison of frozen section consultations: a College of American Pathologists Q-Probes Study of 90,538 cases in 461 institutions. *Arch Pathol Lab Med.* 1996;120:804-809.

8. Zarbo RJ, Schmidt WA, Bachner P, et al. Indications and immediate patient outcomes of pathology intraoperative consultations: College of American Pathologists / Centers for Disease Control and Prevention Outcomes Working Group study. *Arch Pathol Lab Med.* 1996;120:19-25.

9. Sawady J, Berner JJ, Siegler EE. Accuracy of and reasons for frozen sections: a correlative, retrospective study. *Hum Pathol.* 1988;19:1019-1023.

10. Leteurtre E, Leroy X, Pattou F, et al. Why do frozen sections have limited value in encapsulated or minimally invasive follicular carcinoma of thyroid? *Am J Clin Pathol.* 2001;115:370-374.

11. Ferreiro JA, Myers JL, Bostwick DG. Accuracy of frozen section in diagnostic surgical pathology: one year's experience at the Mayo Clinic. *Mod Pathol.* 1995;8:157A.

12. Dankwa EK, Davies JD. Frozen section diagnosis: an audit. *J Clin Pathol.* 1985; 38:1235-1240.

13. Tomaszewski JE, Bear HD, et al. Consensus conference on second opinions in diagnostic anatomic pathology: who, what and when. *Am J Clin Pathol.* 2000;114:329-335.

14. Troxel DB, Sabella JD. Problem areas in pathology practice: uncovered by a review of malpractice claims. *Am J Surg Pathol.* 1994;18:821-831.

15. Renshaw AA. Measuring and reporting errors in surgical pathology: lessons from gynecologic cytology. *Am J Clin Pathol.* 2001:115:338-341.

16. Raab SS, Nakhleh RE, Ruby SG. Patient safety in anatomic pathology: measuring discrepancy frequencies and causes. *Arch Pathol Lab Med.* 2005;129:459-466.

17 Renshaw AA, Cartagena N, Granter SR, Gould EW. Agreement and error rates using blinded review to evaluate surgical pathology of biopsy material. *Am J Clin Pathol.* 2003;119:797-800.

18. Nakhleh RE, Zarbo RJ. Amended reports in surgical pathology and implications for diagnostic error detection and avoidance: a College of American Pathologists Q-Probes study of 1,667,547 accessioned cases in 359 laboratories. *Arch Pathol Lab Med.* 1998;122:303-309.

19. Hilborne LH. Examining amended reports in surgical pathology [editorial]. *Arch Pathol Lab Med.* 1998;122:301-302.

20. Renshaw AA, DiNisco SA, Minter LJ, Cibas ES. A more accurate measure of the false negative rate of Pap smear screening is obtained by determining the false negative rate of the rescreening process. *Cancer.* 1997;81:272-276.

21. Renshaw AA, Pinnar NE, Jiroutek MR, Young ML. Blinded review as a method for quality improvement in surgical pathology. *Arch Pathol Lab Med.* 2002;126:961-963.

22. Safrin RE, Bark CJ. Surgical pathology sign-out: routine review of every case by a second pathologist. *Am J Surg Pathol.* 1993;17:1190-1192.

23. Whitehead ME, Fitzwater JE, Lindley SK, et al. Quality assurance of histopathologic diagnoses: a prospective audit of three thousand cases. *Am J Clin Pathol.* 1984;81:487-491.

24. Lind AC, Bewtra C, Healy JC, Sims KL. Prospective peer review in surgical pathology. *Am J Clin Pathol.* 1995;104:560-566.

25. Ramsay AD, Gallagher PJ. Local audit of surgical pathology: 18 month's experience of peer review-based quality assessment in an English teaching hospital. *Am J Surg Pathol.* 1992;16:476-482.

26. Renshaw AA, Pinnar NE, Jiroutek MR, Young ML. Quantifying the value of in-house consultation in surgical pathology. *Am J Clin Pathol.* 2002;117:751-754.

27. Renshaw AA, Young ML, Jiroutek MR. Many cases need to be reviewed to compare performance in surgical pathology. *Am J Clin Pathol.* 2003;119:388-391.

28. Wakely SL, Baxendine-Jones, Gallagher PJ, Mullee M, Pickering R. Aberrant diagnoses by individual surgical pathologists. *Am J Surg Pathol.* 1998;22:77-82.

29. Renshaw AA. Improved reporting methods for atypia and atypical ductal hyperplasia in breast core needle biopsy specimens: potential for interlaboratory comparisons. *Am J Clin Pathol.* 2001;116:87-91.

30. Nakhleh RE, Azam M, Zarbo RJ. Surgical pathology consultation practices: a College of American Pathologists Q-Probes study in 180 institutions. *Mod Pathol.* 2001;14:229A.

31. Shaw J, Stokes G, Kendall B. Clinical utility of extradepartmental consultations in surgical pathology. *Mod Pathol.* 2001;14:230A.

32. Association of Directors of Anatomic and Surgical Pathology. Consultations in surgical pathology. *Am J Surg Pathol.* 1993;17:743-745.

33. Gupta D, Layfield LJ. Prevalence of inter-institutional anatomic pathology slide review: a survey of current practice. *Am J Surg Pathol.* 2000;24:280-284.

34. Wetherington RW, Cooper HS. Clinical significance of performing and/or repeating immunohistochemistry on patients with previous diagnosis of cancer coming to a National Comprehensive Cancer Center. *Mod Pathol.* 2001;14:230A.

35. Malhotra R, Massimi G, Woda BA. Interinstitutional surgical pathology consultation and its role on patient management. *Mod Pathol.* 1996;9:165A.

36. Kronz JD, Westra WH, Epstein JI. Mandatory second opinion surgical pathology at a large referral hospital. *Cancer.* 1999;86:2426-2435.

37. Abt AB, Abt LG, Olt GJ. The effect of interinstitution anatomic pathology consultation on patient care. Arch Pathol Lab Med. 1995;119:514-517.

38. Weir MM, Jan E, Colgan TJ: Reasons for non-correlating second opinion pathology reviews. *Mod Pathol.* 2001;14:230A.

39. Jacques SM, Qureshi F, Munkarah A, Lawrence WD. Interinstitutional surgical pathology review in gynecologic oncology, I: cancer in endometrial curettings and biopsies. *Int J Gynecol Pathol.* 1998;17:36-41.

40. Kim H, Zelman RJ, Fox MA, et al. Pathology panel for lymphoma clinical studies: a comprehensive analysis of cases accumulated since its inception. *J Natl Cancer Inst.* 1982;68:43-67.

41. Bruner JM, Inouye L, Fuller GN, Langford LA. Diagnostic discrepancies and their clinical impact in a neuropathology referral practice. *Cancer.* 1997;79:796-803.

42. Scott CB, Nelson JS, Farnan NC, et al. Central pathology review in clinical trials for patients with malignant glioma. *Cancer.* 1995;76:307-313.

43. Aldape K, Simmons ML, Davis RL, et al. Discrepancies in diagnoses of neuroepithelial neoplasms: The San Francisco Bay Area Adult Glioma Study. *Cancer.* 2000;88:2342-2349.

44. Santoso JT, Coleman RL, Voet RL, Bernstein SG, Lifshitz S, Miller D. Pathology slide review in gynecologic oncology. *Obstet Gynecol.* 1998;91:730-734.

45. Selman AE, Nieman TH, Fowler JM, Copeland LJ. Quality assurance of second opinion pathology in gynecologic oncology. *Obstet Gynecol.* 1999;94:302-306.

46. McGowan L, Norris JH. The mistaken diagnosis of carcinoma of the ovary. *Surg Gynecol Obstet.* 1991;173:211-215.

47. Harris M, Hartley AL, Blair V, et al. Sarcomas in north west England, I: histopathological peer review. *Br J Cancer.* 1991;64:315-320.

48. Epstein JI, Walsh PC, Sanfilippo F. Clinical and cost impact of second-opinion pathology: review of prostate biopsies prior to radical prostatectomy. *Am J Surg Pathol.* 1996;20:851-857.

49. Cross SS, Feeley KM, Angel CA. The effect of four interventions on the informational content of histopathology reports of resected colorectal carcinomas. *J Clin Pathol.* 1998 Jun;51:481-482.

50. Nakhleh RE, Jones B, Zarbo RJ. Mammographically directed breast biopsies: a College of American Pathologists Q-Probes study of clinical physician expectations and of specimen handling and reporting characteristics in 434 institutions. *Arch Pathol Lab Med.* 1997;121:11-18.

51. Rigby K, Brown SR, Lakin G, Balsitis M, Hosie KB. The use of a proforma improves colorectal cancer pathology reporting. *Ann R Coll Surg Engl.* 1999 Nov;81(6):401-403.

52. Zarbo, RJ. Interinstitutional assessment of colorectal carcinoma surgical pathology report adequacy: a College of American Pathologists Q-Probes study of practice patterns from 532 laboratories and 15,940 reports. *Arch Pathol Lab Med.* 1992;116:1113-1119.

53. Branston LK, Greening S, Newcombe RG, et al. The implementation of guidelines and computerised forms improves the completeness of cancer pathology reporting. *Eur J Cancer.* 2002;38:764-772.

54. Beattie GC, McAdam TK, Elliott S, Sloan JM, Irwin ST. Improvement in quality of colorectal cancer pathology reporting with a standardized proforma: a comparative study. *Colorectal Dis.* 2003;5:558-562.

55. Compton CC, ed. *Reporting on Cancer Specimens: Case Summaries and Background Documentation.* Northfield, Ill: College of American Pathologists; 2005.

56. Phang PT, Law J, Toy E, Speers C, Paltiel C, Coldman AJ. Pathology audit of 1996 and 2000 reporting for rectal cancer in BC. *BC Med J.* 2003;45:319-323.

57. Keating J, Lolohea S, Kenwright D. Pathology reporting of rectal cancer: a national audit. *NZ Med J.* 2003; 116:U514.

58. Ramsay AD. Errors in histopathology reporting: detection and avoidance. *Histopathology.* 1999;34:481-490.

59. Kricker A, Armstrong B, Smith C, et al. An audit of breast cancer pathology reporting in Australia in 1995. *Br J Cancer.* 1999 May;80:563-568

60. Gephardt GN, Baker P. *Lung Carcinoma Surgical Pathology Report Adequacy: Data Analysis and Critique. 91-06A. Q-Probes.* Northfield, Ill: College of American Pathologists; 1992.

61. Gephardt GN, Baker P. Interinstitutional comparison of bladder carcinoma surgical pathology report adequacy: a College of American Pathologists Q-Probes study of 7234 bladder biopsies and curettings in 268 institutions. *Arch Pathol Lab Med.* 1995;119:681-685.

62. Cowan DF, Gray RZ, Campbell B. Validation of the laboratory information system. *Arch Pathol Lab Med.* 1998;122:239-244.

63. Panackal AA, M'ikanatha NM, Tsui FC, et al. Automatic electronic laboratory-based reporting of notifiable infectious diseases at a large health system. *Emerg Infect Dis.* 2002;8:685-691.

64. Howanitz PJ, Cembrowski GS. Postanalytic quality improvement: a College of American Pathologists Q-Probes study of elevated calcium results in 525 institutions. *Arch Pathol Lab Med.* 2000;124:504-510.

65. Zarbo RJ. Quality assessment in anatomic pathology in the cost-conscious era. *Am J Clin Pathol.* 1996;106 (Suppl 1):S3-S10.

66. Zarbo RJ, Gephardt GN, and Howanitz PJ. Intralaboratory timeliness of surgical pathology reports: results of two College of American Pathologists Q-Probes studies of biopsies and complex specimens. *Arch Pathol Lab Med.* 1996;120:234-244.

67. Howanitz JH, Howanitz PJ. Timeliness as a quality attribute and strategy. *Am J Clin Pathol.* 2001;116:311-315.

68. Bachner P, Howanitz PJ, and Lent RW. Quality improvement practices in clinical and anatomic pathology services: a College of American Pathologists Q-Probes study of the program characteristics and performance in 580 institutions. *Am J Clin Pathol.* 1994;102:567-571.

69. Novis DA, Zarbo RJ. Interinstitutional comparison of frozen section turnaround time: a College of American Pathologists Q-Probes study of 32868 frozen sections in 700 hospitals. *Arch Pathol Lab Med.* 1997;121:559-567.

70. Novis DA, Zarbo RJ, and Saladino AJ. Interinstitutional comparison of surgical biopsy diagnosis turnaround time: a College of American Pathologists Q-Probes study of 5384 surgical biopsies in 157 small hospitals. *Arch Pathol Lab Med.* 1998;122:951-956.

71. Smith MT, and Garvin AJ. Anatomic pathology turnaround times: use and abuse. *Am J Clin Pathol.* 1996;106 (Suppl 1):S70-S73.

72. Coard KC and Gibson TN. Turnaround time in the surgical pathology laboratory. *West Indian Med J.* 1999;48:85-87.

73. Nahrig JM, Richter T, Kuhn W, et al. Intraoperative examination of sentinel lymph nodes by ultrarapid immunohistochemistry. *Breast J.* 2003;9:277-281.

74. Soans S, Galindo LM, Garcia FU. Mucin stain on frozen sections: a rapid 3-minute method. *Arch Pathol Lab Med.* 1999;123:378-380.

75. Wendum D, Flejou JF. Quality assessment of intraoperative frozen sections in a teaching hospital: an analysis of 847 consecutive cases. *Ann Pathol.* 2003;23:393-399.

76. Hamoudi AC, Rutledge JC, Novak RW, Hawkins E. Quality improvement approaches: survey of pathologists serving the pediatric patient. *Arch Pathol Lab Med.* 1994;118:165-167.

77. Kazzi JC, Lloyd PJ, Bryant S. Turnaround times for reports on uncomplicated biopsies in five major anatomical pathology laboratories in NSW, Australia. *Pathology.* 1999;31:406-412.

78. Ribe A, Ribalta T, Lledo R, Torras G, Asenjo MA, Cardesa A. Evaluation of turnaround times as a component of quality assurance in surgical pathology. *Int J Qual Health Care.* 1998;10:241-245.

79. Guo A, Li X, Huang W. Timeliness of 5,979 surgical pathology reports. *Zhonghua Bing Li Xue Za Zhi.* 2002;31:530-533.

80. Morales AR, Essenfeld H, Essenfeld E, Duboue MC, Vincek V, Nadji M. Continuous-specimen-flow, high-throughput, 1-hour tissue processing: a system for rapid diagnostic tissue preparation. *Arch Pathol Lab Med.* 2002;126:583-590.

81. Morales AR, Nassiri M, Kanhoush R, Vincek V, Nadji M. Experience with an automated microwave-assisted rapid tissue processing method: validation of histologic quality and impact on the timeliness of diagnostic surgical pathology. *Am J Clin Pathol.* 2004;121:528-536.

82. Zarbo RJ, Nakhleh RE, Walsh M. Customer satisfaction in anatomic pathology: a College of American Pathologists Q-Probes study of 3065 physician surveys from 94 laboratories. *Arch Pathol Lab Med.* 2003;127:23-29.

Quality management in the histology laboratory

Richard W. Brown, MD

Concepts of quality management in the histology laboratory have evolved over the last 25 years. Not surprisingly, emphasis was initially placed on ensuring that laboratories had standard operating procedures and preventive maintenance schedules for equipment, analogous to those used in the clinical laboratory.[1,2] Rickert emphasized the importance of record keeping "in promoting consistently high technical preparations in anatomic pathology" and recommended that records be kept of specimens processed, slides produced, numbers of special stains performed, quality of tissue fixation, and the quality of slides and stains produced.[3] Many of these issues have long been addressed through questions in the College of American Pathologists Laboratory Accreditation Program (LAP) checklists and have become part of routine practice in most clinical histology laboratories.[4]

More recently, emphasis has shifted to ensuring quality of surgical specimen submission, acquisition of proper clinical history, and maintenance of specimen identification and integrity through all steps of the complex process, which includes accessioning, grossing, and the production of a paraffin block and slide.[5,6] The importance of these latter issues has been underscored by media coverage and a recent review of errors in surgical pathology that showed a striking increase in malpractice claims (8% of total claims versus 1.8% in a prior study) from misdiagnoses of malignancy attributable to specimen mix-ups, lost specimens, or extraneous tissue in histologic sections.[7]

This chapter will review basic quality control procedures for histologic sections and special stains, focusing particularly on performance improvement monitors and error reduction strategies to minimize lost specimens, mislabeled slides, and extraneous tissue. The important areas of specimen submission and accessioning are considered separately in chapter 6, and a more extensive discussion of error reduction strategies in anatomic pathology can be found in chapter 4.

Quality control techniques

Daily checklists

Quality control in histology, in contrast to other areas of the clinical laboratory, does not involve numerical values to which upper and lower limits of acceptability can be assigned and monitored. With the exception of temperatures (addressed in the following section), daily quality control involves scrutiny of the grossing and frozen section areas, embedding stations, processors, and automated instruments for staining and coverslipping to ensure that daily maintenance has been performed. One effective means to accomplish this is a daily checklist that can be followed and initialed by the technician assigned to this area of the laboratory. Exhibit 7-1 shows a sample checklist for the frozen section area.

Essential to the success of daily checklists are routine oversight and employee education. The supervisor or senior technologist must review the checklists to ensure that they have been properly completed. The importance of each step in the checklist must be emphasized in the clinical context; review of past errors is an excellent educational tool in this process. Examples of critical errors resulting from seemingly minor infractions of procedure include delays in frozen sections because the cryostat is not at the proper temperature or there is no hematoxylin in the staining rack, or the loss of a run of biopsies due to failure to change alcohols on the processor. The technician must always understand the importance to patient care of even the most mundane tasks.

Temperature and humidity checks

Daily temperature monitoring is an essential quality control measure in histology. As in other areas of the laboratory, refrigerators used for storing unfixed specimens and reagents must be monitored. In the frozen section laboratory, cryostats and rapid cooling devices, like isopentane baths, must be maintained at appropriate temperatures. Tissue can be "cooked," with considerable loss of morphologic detail, by excessive heat at any time in the production of a paraffin section. Therefore, temperatures must be carefully monitored in (1) tissue processors (typically an automated function with alarms), (2) paraffin baths and dispensers in embedding centers, (3) flotation baths at each microtome station, and (4) slide drying ovens and platforms.

Ambient temperature and humidity impact many aspects of the histology laboratory, including proper function of automated instruments, the integrity of chemicals and chemical reactions used in special stains, and storage of slides and blocks. Therefore daily checks of ambient temperature and humidity are required and have been accordingly incorporated into the checklists of the CAP Laboratory Accreditation Program.

Production and review of controls

Controls are used to routinely assess the quality of each product from the histology laboratory, including frozen sections, routine hematoxylin-eosin (H&E) stains, and special stains. Each control must be reviewed before the first product is released from the laboratory. Thus the frozen section control should precede the first frozen section of the day, the H&E control should be reviewed before the first rack of slides is run, and special stain controls should be reviewed before the corresponding patient slide is released from the laboratory. These reviews, at least by a senior technologist and preferably by a pathologist as well, should be documented, either in a dedicated log or incorporated into a daily checklist, as in Exhibit 7-1.

One issue that typically receives little attention is the production of control blocks. The optimal control must address all pertinent issues of histology. For frozen sections, the frozen tissue used for controls should assess cryostat function. Myometrium and skin, which can be obtained fresh from hysterectomy and mastectomy specimens, are excellent for detecting cryostat malfunctions that lead to thick and thin sections and chatter. These tissues will also adequately assess the nuclear detail and staining characteristics needed for optimal frozen section evaluation. Unfortunately, application of this control measure may not be feasible in all laboratory settings because it is difficult to impossible to store frozen tissues without degradation, particularly desiccation and ice crystal artifact, and because of limited availability of excess fresh tissue in some laboratories.

The control blocks used to assess the routine hematoxylin-eosin stain should take into consideration the entire range of tissue processing and should contain tissue elements that allow complete assessment of stain quality. With regard to the former, an optimal control block for the hematoxylin-eosin stain might include a small piece of lung tissue that mimics tissue biopsies; a lymphoid tissue, such as tonsil or spleen, which is effective for monitoring nuclear chromatin staining patterns; and a larger tissue, reflecting the longest processing runs, such as dense breast tissue, colon, skin, or placenta.

In the evaluation of an H&E-stained section, the quality of hematoxylin staining is reflected in the clarity of the chromatin pattern. There should be a range of chromatin staining: epithelial nuclei should demonstrate a well-defined nuclear rim and internal chromatin pattern, while cells with denser nuclei, like lymphocytes and endometrial stromal cells, should show more darkly stained, compact chromatin. The quality of the eosin stain is assessed by the differential staining of red blood cells, smooth muscle, epithelial cell cytoplasm, and collagen. In the optimal stain, there should be three readily discerned shades of eosin. Finally, the contrast between epithelial cell nucleus and cytoplasm should be assessed. Therefore the optimal control block should contain epithelium and a range of stromal components.

Special stains present three unique quality control issues. First, the controls must be carefully selected to reflect the special stain applications that they are intended to control. This is considered in greater detail below. Second, the control materials must be reviewed prior to use to ensure that they contain the structures of interest. This is particularly important in the case of microorganisms. When a series of control sections are cut from a new block, the pathologist should review stains of the first and last sections cut from that block before any of the sections are used to ensure that the structures of interest are demonstrated (so-called "first-last" slide). This review should be documented on a special form used for that purpose.

Third, the laboratory must have in place procedures to ensure that there is no cross-contamination of microorganisms from controls to patient tissues. This is of particular concern with mycobacteria, as the presence of 1 or 2 organisms in a patient tissue may be regarded as diagnostic evidence of infection. Appropriate actions might include using controls that do not contain large numbers of organisms (more prone to floating), cutting controls and patient tissues on separate slides, staining individual slides horizontally rather than in Coplin jars, and, if both are on the same slide, cutting sections for automated stainers such that the flow of reagents is from patient tissue to control. Laboratories may also find it useful to stain a tissue known to be negative (negative control) as surveillance for unexpected cross-contamination from positive controls tissues and from environmental sources such as colonized de-ionized water supplies.

One of the most common failures of quality control in histology is the lack of appropriate special stain controls. There are two basic principles that must be considered: (1) neoplastic tissues are biochemically different than normal tissue and (2) appropriate staining of one tissue element does not guarantee accurate staining of others for which the same stain is used. For example, the typical target of a mucicarmine stain is an adenocarcinoma, which contains much less mucin than normal bowel. Thus, if one wishes to ensure adequate sensitivity for detecting mucin in adenocarcinoma, the most appropriate control would be an adenocarcinoma. Similarly, if one is using a trichrome stain to identify smooth muscle, a section of liver with adequate staining of the collagen will do little to ensure that smooth muscle is staining appropriately. The sensitivity of silver stains for organisms differs. Therefore, if a Gomori methenamine silver stain is used to identify both fungi and *Pneumocystis* organisms, examples of both must be included in the control block. Including tissues that address the most common applications in a single, multi-tissue control block is an efficient way to produce useful controls. Additional examples are listed as follows.

Special stain controls

Stain	Application	Control
Alcian blue	Tumoral mucin	Adenocarcinoma
	Barrett's metaplasia	Intestinal metaplasia
	Stromal mucin	Umbilical cord
Elastin	Medial degeneration in atherosclerosis	Atherosclerotic aorta
	Identification of pleural/vascular invasion	Lung
Fontana-Masson	Pigmented fungi	Fungal sinusitis - mucin
	Neuroendocrine cells	Carcinoid
	Melanin	Malignant melanoma
Gram (All blocks should contain + and -)	Gram positive	*Clostridium* or *Streptococcus*
	Gram negative	*E. coli* or *Pseudomonas*
PAS	Basement membrane	Kidney
	Fungus	Candida spp.
	Glycogen	Liver
PAS with diastase	Alpha-1-antitrypsin	Liver
	Tumoral mucin	Adenocarcinoma
Reticulin	Tumor architecture	Paraganglioma
	Liver biopsy	Cirrhotic liver
	Hematopoietic tissues	Spleen
Trichrome	Smooth muscle vs collagen	Leiomyoma
	Liver biopsy	Cirrhotic liver

A final consideration for special stain controls is that fixation and processing may have a major impact on the sensitivity of the procedure. Therefore, whenever possible, controls should be obtained from archival tissues of the laboratory unless it is impossible to obtain appropriate tissue, as in the case of rare microorganisms. Two creative solutions to obtaining controls include growing microorganisms in fresh tissue, such as placenta, and obtaining wet tumor tissue from neighboring laboratories for in-house processing.

External quality assessment

The utility of a program by which histology laboratories could obtain an objective assessment of slide quality from an external source has been recognized since the publication in 1982 of a study from Wales in which slides prepared from standard material were submitted for external evaluation using a very basic evaluation scheme that ranged from excellent to unsatisfactory.[8] A successful national external quality assessment program (NEQAS) has been in place in the United Kingdom for years.

Until recently, no comparable program was available in the United States. HistoQIP, a recently developed joint program of the College of American Pathologists and the National Society for Histotechnology, now offers an external assessment of slide staining quality. Each laboratory is asked to submit a designated stain using tissue processed in that laboratory and the routine laboratory staining protocol. Currently, two hematoxylin-eosin stains, two special stains, and one immunohistochemical stain per challenge are reviewed by experienced evaluators, both histotechnologists and pathologists, using standardized criteria for evaluation. The quality score can be benchmarked against other laboratories in the program using frequency distribution data. Educational materials are also provided, and continuing education credits can be obtained based on review of these materials.

Performance improvement monitors in histology

Turnaround times

A basic performance improvement monitor throughout anatomic pathology is turnaround time. In histology, it is possible to separately monitor the turnaround time for routine histologic sections, additional sections (ie, "recuts," levels), and special stains. There are two approaches that can be used to track turnaround time in histology. The first is to use specific time "stamps" through the laboratory information system. This approach requires an entry at the time tissue blocks are submitted or a special request is made, and an entry when the slides are released from the laboratory. With this approach, the actual turnaround time in hours can be specifically determined and trended.

The second approach, providing a simpler and more global view, is to predetermine specific cutoff points with the pathologist consumers of the laboratory, and then track the frequency with which the contracted deadline is met. For example, there could be an agreement that for all tissues grossed on day 1, 90% of the biopsy slides would be released by 9 AM on day 2, and 90% of the routine surgical cases would be available by 1 PM. For special stains and additional sections, the agreed upon expectation may be that any requests submitted by 11 AM would be completed the same day. The difficulty with this approach is that it may require a global assessment of "completion" by the technician assigned to release the slides and manual recording of those data, a system that is both labor intensive and error prone.

Quality of histologic sections

Assessing histologic section quality requires the cooperation of all pathologists receiving histologic preparations from the laboratory, and the supervisor and medical director must work together to ensure that pathologist input is meaningful and consistent. In the assessment of slide quality for performance improvement, it is important to distinguish slides that are less than optimal from those in which defects significantly detract from the pathologist's ability to make a histopathologic diagnosis. Additionally, pathologists should be encouraged to indicate the specific problems encountered rather than providing a global assessment of "poor."

A quality assessment form, as illustrated in Exhibit 7-2, can be useful in ensuring pathologist cooperation. In this system, pathologists are instructed to enumerate problems using coded comments and individual case numbers. This form assists the histology laboratory in documenting individual corrective action, in compiling summary reports by defect, and in detecting trends.[9] In addition, however, the pathologist should be asked to make a global assessment. "Unacceptable" quality is defined as one or more errors in processing, microtomy, or staining that compromise diagnosis. The frequency of "unacceptable" quality can then be monitored as a global quality management issue with appropriate threshold, as this directly impacts patient care. A sample quality assessment summary report is provided in Exhibit 7-3.

"Lost" specimens

The comprehensive "Recommendations on quality control and quality assurance in surgical pathology and autopsy pathology," published in 1991 by the members of the Association of Directors of Anatomic and Surgical Pathology (ADASP),[5] defined a lost specimen as "the irretrievable loss of a surgical pathology specimen that has occurred after the case has been accessioned in the laboratory and that prevents an adequate pathologic examination of that specimen." The acceptable threshold for these events, which would include both loss of gross tissue and processing events, was defined by ADASP as 1 in 3000 cases.

Trending of cases in which there has been a partial or complete irretrievable loss of tissue is an important monitor for histology laboratories. It is insufficient, however, to only gather data. Each case should be investigated and the results of that investigation reported to the submitting physician and, when appropriate, to hospital risk management. One method of investigation is the failure modes effects analysis, as described below.

A specimen may be lost at any of multiple steps in the histology process. At the time of grossing, the tissue or an entire tissue cassette may be left on a paper towel and inadvertently discarded. Selection of the wrong cassette type (large tissue cassette for small biopsies), failure to properly wrap small tissues, or failure to completely close cassettes may result in tissue floating away during processing. Tissue may be missed or detached from forceps during the embedding process. Tissue may be cut away at the time of frozen section or, more rarely, during sectioning of the paraffin block. Finally, tissue blocks may be lost during the process of transportation from a peripheral site to a core laboratory.

One useful step to minimize these occurrences is careful use of a histopathology worksheet, as shown in Exhibit 7-4. The essential steps in specimen tracking that should be incorporated into standard operating procedures and employee training are as follows.

1. The pathologist or grossing assistant should always compare the labeling of each cassette with the requisition and specimen container. The cassette is inspected to ensure that tissue is present in the cassette before it is closed. The case number, specimen, and specific identifiers of each cassette submitted (eg, 1A-1C) are recorded in the appropriate columns on the histology worksheet.

2. If the cassettes are being sent from a remote location to a core laboratory, the person sending the cassettes should confirm that all submitted blocks are present in the secondary container being transported and should document this review by initialing in the "cassette check" column of the worksheet. The technician loading the processor at the core laboratory should

then check each cassette against the worksheet a second time to ensure that all cassettes are being loaded and that the labeling of the cassettes matches that of the worksheet. This individual then places their initials in the "core check" column.

3. The technician organizing the paraffin blocks following processing and embedding checks the blocks against the worksheet, again confirming that all blocks submitted are present and contain tissue, and records their initials in the "block" column.

Essential to the success of this process is immediate notification of the pathologist or supervisor and prompt investigation at the time an error is discovered. The laboratory should maintain a standard procedure for the immediate investigation of missing tissue/cassettes. Elements of this investigation include:

- Inspecting trash from the grossing area, when possible, to determine if a cassette or tissue was inadvertently discarded.
- Examining the original specimen container and any secondary transportation buckets for missing cassettes. If a frozen section block is missing, the cryostat should be examined.
- Reviewing the gross description to determine if the blocks were recorded on the worksheet in error (ie, worksheet states A1-A5, blocks A1-A4 received, gross description confirms only blocks A1-A4 were submitted).
- Examining all materials from the embedding centers, including the original cassette and lid, biopsy bags, and filter papers, if tissue is missing from the paraffin block, as identified at the time of block check or subsequently by the reviewing pathologist.

Floatation errors

A floatation error is one in which the wrong tissue has been picked up on the microscopic section. This can be due to mislabeling of the slides or the failure of the technician to check the slide against the block when cutting. The former can be largely eliminated by the use of automated slide labelers, which receive input directly from the laboratory information system. Thus each block that is entered into the workload triggers one or more corresponding slides. Alternately, a single individual working directly from the histopathology worksheet (see Exhibit 7-4) should label the slides. Labeling of additional slides out of sequence by the technician at the time of cutting should be discouraged.

There are three principle strategies that can be used to minimize floatation errors. First, technicians should be instructed to handle the slides and blocks from only one case at a time. Second, if possible the same technician should not cut like cases consecutively. That is, one person should not be assigned to cut a series of placentas or all of the needle biopsies. Like tissues should be distributed among multiple technicians to the greatest extent possible. This strategy can be augmented by a policy that states two of the same type of tissue should not be accessioned consecutively. Obviously, these strategies cannot apply to laboratories in which all specimens are similar (eg, prostate needle and skin biopsies).

The third and perhaps most important error identification and reduction procedure is at the time of slide release, often referred to as "sign-out." Optimally, a technician experienced in tissue morphology should release the slides. This technician should match all slides against the histopathology worksheet (Exhibit 7-4), taking care to ensure that both the number of slides and the designation match those of the submitted blocks. In addition, this individual should verify that that the tissue appears consistent from block to block and is consistent with the tissue designation on the worksheet. The most desirable process is to match the slides against the blocks at the time of sign-out to ensure that all tissue in the block is present in the section; however, in large laboratories this is usually not possible. Laboratories should consider, however, adopting this practice at least for nongastrointestinal biopsy specimens.

The trending of floatation errors is one of the most important quality monitors in histology. While reduction in the absolute numbers of errors is an important performance improvement initiative, the potential consequence is grave, and therefore each occurrence should be individually investigated and the results of the investigation recorded. Essential to successful investigation is a mechanism by which the technician cutting a particular case can be identified. Some laboratories require the technician to initial all cases cut. Recurrent errors by one technician should be followed with counseling and, if unsuccessful, retraining efforts to include documented educational activities, structured microtomy practice under direct supervision, and additional competency assessment before allowing the employee to return to unsupervised work. Such efforts demonstrate a process-based educational approach to resolving employee performance problems while also contributing to error reduction. As with lost specimens, recurrent events should also trigger a failure mode effects analysis to scrutinize the cutting process for effects of fatigue and interruptions as well as operational issues, like the way in which labeled slides and blocks are presented to the technician.

Extraneous tissue

Small pieces of tissue that arise from a source other than the case under examination, or "floaters," can be seen in a single section on a slide or can be embedded in the paraffin block. Extraneous tissue present in only one section is usually attributable to cross-contamination in the process of microtomy or staining. When present in every section on a slide, the extraneous tissue is embedded in the block, which is attributed to cross-contamination during grossing, processing, or embedding. Identification of extraneous tissue by the pathologist can be tracked using the form in Exhibit 7-2, and numbers of occurrences per total tissue blocks or slides can be aggregated as a useful performance improvement monitor. Extraneous tissue can lead to misdiagnosis, thus representing a sometimes critical process error, warranting continuous evaluation. Furthermore, this is one of the few histology monitors for which an external benchmark exists.

In 1994, participants in the Q-Probes program of the College of American Pathologists were asked to perform a review of microscopic sections for extraneous tissue and report these occurrences. In this study of 275 laboratories, the average rate of occurrence on prospective slide review and the 50th percentile of occurrence rate for participant laboratories were 0.6% and 0.31% of slides, 0.8% and 0.43% of blocks, and 1.2% and 0.69% of specimens.[10] Laboratories with occurrence rates higher than the median figures should examine processes to establish mechanisms for improvement.

There are no published studies that address the most common causes of tissue contaminants; however, prudent laboratory practice and anecdotal experience suggest the following steps that can be taken to reduce its frequency.

- All instruments used in grossing, including forceps, scalpels, and scissors, should be rigorously cleaned after every case.

- Small biopsies should be grossed without instruments whenever possible, for example by pouring the contents of the formalin container directly through an embedding bag or filter paper within a funnel.

- Specimens containing small fragments should be processed with precautions to minimize carry-over, such as the use of biopsy cassettes, embedding bags, papers or sponges. Tissues commonly associated with floaters include villous adenomas of the colon, testicular germ cell tumors, products of conception, bone marrow clot sections, and transurethral resection of bladder tumor. All cassettes from such cases should be carefully inspected for external contaminants and/or wiped before being placed into common formalin containers.

- Cassettes containing tissues with high potential for contamination (eg, placentas) should be segregated during primary fixation and, when possible, in the tissue processors.

- Embedding forceps must be carefully cleansed of paraffin after every case.

- Policies should be developed that address pieces of tissue encountered away from the main specimen (eg, outside the embedding bag/paper, on the outside of the cassette). These should never be added automatically to the case being embedded but instead should be separately embedded and labeled as a "floater" for microscopic review by the pathologist.

- Microtome blades should be carefully cleansed of residual paraffin fragments between tissue blocks.

- Flotation baths at microtome stations should be frequently cleaned, particularly following any poorly processed tissue that "explodes" on the water bath surface.

- Stains should be changed frequently on a predetermined schedule, and there should be a policy by which the stains are visually inspected or tested for the presence of "floaters" using blank slides.

Fortunately, the data from the Q-Probes study would suggest that extraneous tissue rarely causes diagnostic difficulty. In that study, only 0.4% of the extraneous tissues identified were judged to cause severe diagnostic difficulty, while 90.1% caused no difficulty at all. Furthermore, only 12.7% of the extraneous tissues identified were neoplastic. Despite these encouraging data, the disastrous consequences of an erroneous malignant diagnosis due to the presence of an extraneous tissue mandate careful scrutiny of practices. Additionally, laboratories are encouraged to develop policies and procedures for the investigation, labeling/removal, and documentation of extraneous tissue identified in slides and blocks.

Assessing pathologist satisfaction

Routine assessment of pathologist satisfaction can serve as a useful performance improvement initiative, particularly when compared with results of routine monitoring of slide quality (see Exhibit 7-3). Surveys are most useful in laboratories serving multiple pathologists, particularly in settings where they are at multiple sites. In performance assessments surveys, pathologists could be asked to rate on a scale of 1 to 5 or 1 to 10 their level of satisfaction with:

- Quality and turnaround times for routine slides (with further division of the quality section, if desired, into fixation/processing, embedding, staining, and coverslipping)
- Quality and turnaround times for recuts and special stains
- Accuracy and quality of slide and block labeling
- Accuracy of verbal order transcription and telephone etiquette of laboratory personnel (if applicable)
- Response of laboratory personnel to complaints and verbal requests
- Availability of laboratory personnel, particularly supervisory level, for questions and consultation

Ideally, pathologist surveys are distributed at established intervals (eg, yearly) that allow for linear assessment of quality and the results of interval performance improvement initiatives.

Conducting a failure mode effects analysis in histology

The failure mode effects analysis (FMEA) is a technique for assessing a complex system for potential errors initially designed in the manufacturing industry.[11] The FMEA is ideally suited to the histology laboratory as the production of a histologic section is a complex, multi-step, and potentially error-prone process. The FMEA can be used following an error to assess the severity, effect, and potential for recurrence. In this mode, the process for producing a slide can then be re-designed to minimize the potential for recurrence. Alternately, the FMEA can be used in the initial design of a laboratory and its processes to identify every step at which an error may occur and the kind of errors that can occur. By using this analytical technique, the process can be designed initially to be ideally error-free. In addition, steps can be built into the system by which errors can be rapidly detected and addressed.

The first step in conducting a FMEA is to determine each step in the process. Then for each step the potential failure mode(s), the causes and effects are established. Finally, a ranking is assigned for each failure mode that assesses (1) severity, (2) the probability of occurrence, and (3) the probability of detection. For example, an error with a remote probability of occurrence would be assigned a value of 1, while a failure mode with an almost certain probability of occurrence is assigned a value of 10. Severity rankings range from minor events with minimal effect on the system (score 1), to critical or catastrophic events (score 10). Errors that can be detected easily and their effects averted are assigned a score of 1; the least detectable events are assigned the highest score. These three scores are then multiplied to obtain the risk priority number, or "RPN." The failure modes with the highest RPN should be targeted as the highest priority for intervention. An example from histology follows.

Process step	Cutting a section from a designated paraffin block onto the corresponding slide
Potential failure mode	The wrong slide is selected
Potential effect	The slide is erroneously interpreted by the pathologist
Potential cause	Slides from more than one case are lined up side by side
Potential cause	The slides are arranged out of order
Potential cause	The technician does not match the slide and block before picking up the section
Severity	4 (if within a case), 10 (out of 10) if two cases are mixed
Occurrence	7 (a likely event)
Detection	8 (out of 10) assuming that no slide-to-block matching step is in place at sign-out
RPN	256

This step results in a high RPN and should be targeted for system improvement. The result of specific interventions should be that the occurrence happens less frequently and is more detectable. Interventions that would accomplish these goals in the example above would include retraining of technicians to match the slide and block for every block before picking up the section, and establishing a slide-block matching procedure at the time of slide sign-out.

This discussion is a very simplified view of a complex analysis. In some cases, a failure mode effect analysis in histology will require the assistance of an individual specifically trained in this technique as part of a "Six Sigma" program.[12] With the endorsement of these techniques by the Joint Commission on Accreditation of Healthcare Organizations (JCAHO), these individuals specifically trained in error reduction strategies, commonly known as "black belts" and "green belts," are now available in many health care institutions.

Exhibit 7-1. Frozen section area documentation

FROZEN SECTION AREA DOCUMENTATION

Month	1	2	3	4	5	6	7	8	9	10	11	12	13	14	15	16	17	18	19	20	21	22	23	24	25	26	27	28	29	30	31
Daily:																															
Temperature logs																															
address unlabeled specimens																															
clean used cryostats																															
cut control block																															
address staining solutions																															
stain control slide																															
supply inventory																															
frozen gross set-up																															
computer entry, print labels																															
clean and disinfect area																															
Weekly defrost & decontaminate:																															
Leica 1800																															
Leica 1850																															

See policy and procedure manual for complete instructions
See manufacturer manual for cryostat malfunction
Documentation completed Monday through Friday

Exhibit 7-2. Histology quality improvement

Date: _____

If slides are unacceptable, please list case, stain, and problem, using appropriate codes.

Case #	Stain	Problem	Case #	Stain	Problem

Comments: _____

_____

_____

Reviewed by Pathologist: _____

Problem Codes

Fixation / Processing	Microtomy	Staining / Coverslipping
F1 Poor/incomplete fixation	M1 Knife lines	S1 Nuclear too dark/muddy
F2 Inadequate processing	M2 Chatter	S2 Nuclear stain too light
F3 Cell shrinkage	M3 Cracked/torn section	S3 Cytoplasmic/counterstain too light
F4 Incorrect orientation	M4 Section too thick	S4 Cytoplasmic/counterstain too dark
F5 Pigment (formalin, mercury)	M5 Folds	S5 Uneven staining
F6 Excessive/inadequate decalcification	M6 Extraneous tissue Floaters/debris	S6 Section cloudy
	M7 Incomplete section	S7 Desired structures overstained
		S8 Desired structures understained
		S9 Nonspecific background/precipitate
		S10 Air bubble
		S11 Excessive mounting media
		S12 Excessive digestion/retrieval

Comments and Corrective Action: _____

_____

_____

Reviewed by: _____ Date: _____

Exhibit 7-3. Quality assurance quarterly indicators

3rd Quarter 2004-2005

Facility Address   Department Name
                                                                    Histology

Indicator	Routine histology to include processing, cutting, and H&E stains.
Start date	January 2005
Rationale	Accurate anatomic pathology diagnosis requires the best possible quality of histologic preparation.
Responsible party	Histology supervisor
Goal	To have a performance rating of no less 98%. To identify areas for improvement.
Data source	Histology Quality Improvement form, quality assurance data.
Sample	All Quality Improvement forms returned by pathologists or completed by histology personnel in response to verbal comments or requests for repeat are reviewed. A total slide count is gathered in a CCL program from Cerner.
Observations	A total of 51 QI forms were reviewed. No score fell below 98%. Top five problems reported were: Poor fixation - 12, inadequate processing - 8, incomplete section -5, incorrect labeling and poor cutting - 5
Evaluation	Each problem is addressed as it is noted. The slides are reviewed as available. Corrective action is documented on the QI form.
Action	Poor fixation: reviewed fixation with all facilities. Processing problems addressed with group effort to include suggestions from manufacturer. Embedding and cutting procedures and techniques reviewed with staff. Filing and labeling procedures reviewed, QC stressed. Continue to review.

Reviewed by: _____   Date: _____

Reviewed by: _____   Date: _____

Reviewed by: _____   Date: _____

Exhibit 7-4. Histopathology worksheet

Date: _____

Pathologist: _____

CAS ✔	CORE ✔	CASE #	SPECIMEN	LABELED CASSETTES	HSE	RTN	LRG	OV	BLK	COMMENT	SLI

References

1. Sheehan DC, Hrapchak BB. *Theory and Practice of Histotechnology.* 2nd ed. St. Louis, Mo: Mosby; 1980: 406-439.

2. Howanitz PT. Quality assurance measurements in departments of pathology and laboratory medicine. *Arch Pathol Lab Med.* 1990;114:1131-1135.

3. Rickert RR. Quality assurance goals in surgical pathology. *Arch Pathol Lab Med.* 1990;114:1157-1162.

4. College of American Pathologists Commission on Laboratory Accreditation. *Anatomic Pathology Checklist.* Northfield, Ill: College of American Pathologists; 2004.

5. Association of Directors of Anatomic and Surgical Pathology. Recommendations on quality control and quality assurance in surgical pathology and autopsy pathology. *Am J Surg Pathol.* 1991;15:1007-1009.

6. Bancroft J, Gamble M. *Theory and Practice of Histological Techniques.* London: Harcourt; 2002.

7. Troxel DB. Error in surgical pathology. *Am J Surg Pathol.* 2004;28:1092-1095.

8. Barr WT, Williams ED. Value of external quality assessment of the technical aspects of histopathology. *J Clin Pathol.* 1982;35:1050-1056.

9. Larsen PA, Bartlett LM, Bozzo PD. Quality improvement monitors for histologic surgical preparations. *J Histotechnol.* 2004;27:141-144.

10. Gephardt GN, Zarbo RJ. Extraneous tissue in surgical pathology: a College of American Pathologists Q-Probes study in 275 laboratories. *Arch Pathol Lab Med.* 1996;120:1009-1014.

11. Krouwer JS. An improved failure mode effects analysis for hospitals. *Arch Pathol Lab Med.* 2004;128:663-667.

12. Nevalainen D, Berte L, Kraft C, Leigh E, Picaso L, Morgan T. Evaluating laboratory performance on quality indicators with the six sigma scale. *Arch Pathol Lab Med.* 2000;124:516-519.

Quality management in immunohistochemistry

Richard W. Brown, MD

Overview

Diagnostic immunohistochemistry is an integral part of surgical pathology. While used most often to determine cell lineage, immunohistochemistry is emerging as an increasingly important tool in the assessment of prognosis and determination of therapeutic modalities.

While immunohistochemistry is thought of as an analytic procedure, quality management extends beyond the analytic phase and involves all phases of the test cycle.[1-3] In the preanalytical phase, the quality of tissue handling, fixation, and processing ultimately affects the quality of the immunohistochemical staining. In the analytical phase, the major quality issues are reproducible and validated procedures, daily quality control, and interpretation, including external quality assessment. The challenge in the postanalytical phase is accurate and clear reporting of stain results. This chapter will review each of these issues in detail and conclude with suggested quality assurance monitors for the immunohistochemistry laboratory. A discussion of immunohistochemical procedures is beyond the scope of this chapter; further details may be found in standard textbooks on this subject.[3,4]

Preanalytical phase

Tissue fixation and processing

Several authors have suggested that the ultimate goal in immunohistochemistry is standardization.[3,5-7] Ideally, all laboratories would use well-characterized validated primary antibodies, a standard detection system manufactured using rigorous quality control, and automated staining protocols. While this would, in theory, achieve reproducible results that could be meaningfully compared across laboratories, the major obstacle remains the variability inherent in tissue handling.

Antigens are proteins, subject to degradation and conformational alteration. In the early years of immunohistochemistry, the most significant issue was the loss of antigen immunoreactivity due to prolonged formalin fixation. This problem has been largely eliminated by heat induced antigen retrieval, in which incubation of tissue sections in buffer solution heated to the boiling point appears to reverse the configurational changes and other deleterious effects to antigenic sites that are induced by formalin fixation and paraffin tissue processing.[8] What cannot be reversed, however, is loss of antigenicity due to protein degradation.

In order to achieve reproducible immunohistochemical staining, it is essential that tissue sections submitted for processing are thin (less than 3 mm), small (ideally less than 2 x 2 cm), and adequately fixed in formalin. The tissue should be trimmed fresh, ideally within 30 minutes of receipt, to minimize antigen degradation and diffusion of cytoplasmic proteins out of the cell (eg, kappa/lambda, thyroglobulin) due to loss of cell membrane integrity. If there will be significant delay, an alternate approach is to submit a single well-trimmed block of tumor in advance of the remaining dissection.

The time required for adequate fixation varies with the tissue type and size; however, in general, large blocks of excised tumor tissue should be fixed for 12 to 24 hours before processing. If there is insufficient primary fixation, the tissue becomes primarily fixed in alcohol on the processor. Since the mechanism of formalin fixation is the formation of cross-links between proteins, while alcohol fixation results in protein coagulation, differential fixation in alcohol and formalin results in uneven staining of large tissue. This represents one of the most significant sources of variability in immunohistochemistry today.[9] Depending on the antigen and the form of antigen retrieval employed, uneven staining may be loss of staining centrally with enhancement of the peripheral rim of tissue or the reverse with increased staining centrally. Inadequate fixation and processing will also be suggested by tissue detachment centrally during heat induced antigen retrieval. It is possible to decrease some of these deleterious effects by reversing the tissue processing procedure and post-fixing the tissue before reprocessing. Post-fixation in zinc formalin has been shown to be particularly effective in enhancing the antigenicity of poorly fixed lymphoid tissue.[10]

Analytical phase

Standardization and procedures

Standard well-documented procedures are an essential element of quality management in the immunohistochemistry laboratory. The goal of these procedures is to minimize variability to the greatest extent possible. Interinstitutional studies have shown that the most important tools in achieving reproducible results are the routine application of an antigen retrieval step; use of quality controlled, prepackaged detection systems; and the use of automation.[7,11-13] Antigen retrieval, particularly the incubation of tissue sections in preheated buffer, reduces considerably the inherent variation in antigen preservation that results from tissue handling and processing. Inadequate antigen retrieval has been documented as the single most common cause of nonreproducible staining for estrogen and progesterone receptors.[14,15]

Automation can greatly reduce the inevitable variability that occurs with the manual application and timed incubation of multiple immunohistochemical reagents. Additionally, the use of prediluted antibodies may be helpful in some laboratories, as this too will reduce the variability and potential for error that exists in the manual dilution of concentrated antibodies. However, the use of prediluted preparations should never be at the expense of optimal staining; it is not always possible to adjust the staining protocol sufficiently to achieve optimal staining of a given laboratory's tissue with prediluted reagents.

There are two elements that must be addressed in written laboratory procedures to assure optimal stain quality. First, the clone, optimal dilution, antigen retrieval technique, detection system (if nonstandard), specificity, expected pattern of immunoreactivity, and recommended control tissue must be written for each primary antibody in use.

Second, assuming the laboratory's routine staining protocol is for formalin-fixed, paraffin-embedded tissue, any departure from the use of standard tissue sections must be addressed by appropriate procedural modifications and documented in the laboratory procedure manual. Possible exceptions include use of other fixatives, such as zinc formalin for lymphoid tissues or alcoholic formalin for breast; frozen section or cytologic preparations (cytospins, smears, alcohol-fixed cell blocks); and decalcification, including bone marrow core biopsies. It is possible that procedural modifications are not required; however, in this case the laboratory must document appropriate staining of these alternate specimens in a validation study before routine clinical use.

Antibody evaluation and validation

The performance characteristics of each new antibody introduced into the immunohistochemistry laboratory must be appropriately validated before the antibody is placed into clinical use. The initial goal is to establish the optimal titration, detection system, and antigen retrieval protocol. Once the antibody is optimized, it must be tested on laboratory tissues in order to determine the sensitivity and specificity. The scope of the validation is at the discretion of the laboratory director and will vary with the antibody. For a well-characterized antibody with a limited spectrum of antigenic targets, like chromogranin or prostate specific antigen, the validation can be limited. A panel of 10 positive and 10 negative neoplasms would be sufficient in this setting.[16] For an antibody that is not well characterized and/or has a wide range of reported reactivity, a more extensive validation is necessary. The number of tissues tested should in this circumstance be large enough to determine whether the staining profile matches that previously described. The staining profile may be obtained from the primary literature or sources such as ImmunoQuery, a website developed by Dr. Dennis Frisman, in which published data are aggregated.

A simple approach to evaluation and validation of a concentrated antibody preparation is summarized in stepwise fashion below. If a prediluted preparation is being evaluated, the first two steps may be omitted. Careful records of this validation should be maintained.

Step 1. Obtain the optimal antibody titer and antigen retrieval protocol from the manufacturer's specification sheet, if available. If the antibody is an analyte-specific reagent for which no information is reported, these data must be obtained from the published literature.

Step 2. Test the antibody at the recommended dilution and one dilution on either side (eg, 1:40, 1:80, 1:160) using tissues known to possess and lack the target antigen. This is most efficiently performed using sections of a tissue block containing multiple samples fixed and processed the same as regular patient samples. Use the standard laboratory detection system and the recommended antigen retrieval protocol. If none of these dilutions is optimal, as defined by intense specific staining in the appropriate pattern in the absence of nonspecific staining, it may be necessary to extend the dilution series into more concentrated or dilute preparations.

Step 3. Using the optimal titer obtained in Step 2 or the prediluted antibody, stain the same series of positive and negative tissues using a variety of antigen retrieval techniques. For example, the panel could include enzyme treatment (eg, ficin, pepsin, proprietary protease), heat induced antigen retrieval using citrate buffer pH6 and a high pH buffer, and enzyme plus nonenzymatic retrieval. Depending on the results, it may be necessary to adjust the titer.

If there is little difference in retrieval methods, it is most practical to use the "standard" protocol for the laboratory. If none of these methods yield intense specific staining in the absence of nonspecific staining, it may be necessary in rare instances to test a different method that employs increased incubation times or a different detection system, such as enhanced sensitivity polymer.

Step 4. Test a larger series of positive and negative tissues, a minimum of 10 each, until the sensitivity and specificity of the technique are determined to be adequate. Precision must also be established by running serial sections of one or more positive control(s) on different days, typically 10 consecutive runs. There should be little to no variation in staining.

Finally, it is best practice to assure that the antibody performance remains stable over time. If an antibody is used frequently and a single pathologist reviews all controls, this can be accomplished by daily quality control procedures. Laboratories in which an antibody is infrequently requested may wish to use a surveillance program, by periodically running a control or expected positive tissue sample, in order to exclude unexpected deterioration in antibody performance. Audit systems by

Table 8-1. Key parameters that may have an adverse effect on staining quality

Monitor	Potential Adverse Effect
Temperature of processors, embedding centers, and slide drying apparatus	Antigen degradation due to excessive heat
pH of antigen retrieval solution	Decreased immunoreactivity due to incorrect pH
Temperature of antigen retrieval solution/chamber	Failure to reach the optimal temperature (typically less than optimal staining)
Checklist for automated instrument set-up	Selection of incorrect protocol or failure to apply correct reagents results in absence of desired immunoreactivity
Reagent expiration dates	Use of reagents beyond the manufacturer's expiration date may result in inconsistent staining

which slides are reviewed retrospectively and scored for consistency have also been described and may be useful in situations where controls are reviewed by multiple pathologists.[17]

Validation of new reagent lots

Each new reagent lot must be validated before it is used in clinical assays; however, this validation is considerably easier than initial validation. For an established primary antibody that is performing well, the laboratory need only stain a small series of tissues, including the routine positive and negative tissue controls, at the same dilution using the lot of antibody currently in use and the new lot of reagent. Addition of a serial dilution of the new lot on either side may be useful to further define the sensitivity and specificity of the lot. If there is essentially equivalent staining, the new lot is accepted. A sample form for recording this validation is found in Exhibit 8-1. For new lots of detection system reagents, a similar side-by-side comparison of the old and new lots should be performed and recorded using a series of monoclonal and polyclonal primary antibodies that optimally test the sensitivity and specificity of the detection system. For example, a validation set might include cyclin D1 and CD15, antibodies that require optimal sensitivity, and polyclonal antibodies to kappa/lambda and thyroglobulin to assess the degree to which the new reagents minimize nonspecific staining and optimize the signal-to-noise ratio. In laboratories performing predictive markers (eg, ER, HER2/*neu*), these should be included as well to ensure consistent staining from lot to lot.

Routine quality control

As in any area of the laboratory, routine quality control measures are essential to the success of an immunohistochemical stain. Key parameters that may adversely affect the staining quality and thus require careful monitoring are listed in Table 8-1.

Daily controls

Careful selection and rigorous review of controls is an essential quality assurance measure in the immunohistochemistry laboratory. The size and scope of the laboratory determines the manner in which controls are reviewed. Thus the optimal mechanism must be determined by the laboratory director; however, daily review of all slides by a single pathologist skilled in the interpretation of immunohistochemical stains allows early detection of subtle shifts and trends in staining intensity or pattern. In laboratories that use working solutions of concentrated antibodies, it is not unusual to see a gradual decline in staining with time. When controls are serially reviewed by one observer, this trend becomes evident before unsatisfactory staining occurs.

Positive tissue controls

Positive tissue controls assess the sensitivity of the primary antibody and should be performed for each antibody on a run. When feasible, including the positive control on the same slide as the patient tissue ensures that the appropriate antibody and all elements of the detection system were unequivocally applied to that slide. If the positive control tissue is on a separate slide, the laboratory must ensure that this section receives identical slide drying, antigen retrieval, and staining. In staining racks that employ capillary gap, the control slide should be paired with the patient tissue.

Tissues selected for positive tissue controls should (1) reflect the range of antigen density that may be found in patient samples, (2) include the major tumors in which the target antigens are found, and (3) consist of tissue fixed and processed similarly to the patient tissue, ideally within the same laboratory. Appropriate controls for a representative sample of commonly applied antibodies are listed in Exhibit 8-2.

Regarding the need for controls at several levels of staining intensity, a recent quality assurance study in the United Kingdom demonstrated that the best performing laboratories in an interinstitutional review of staining for prostate specific antigen were those in which the control included both well-differentiated and poorly-differentiated prostate cancer.[18] In general, failure to include poorly-differentiated tumors may result in a method that is not sufficiently sensitive to detect the reduced antigen expression seen in high-grade malignant tumors. Similarly, due to the differences in antigen density between normal tissue and neoplasms, laboratories should avoid exclusive use of normal tissues for controls. The use of controls containing antigen at three levels (negative, weakly/moderately positive, strongly positive) is particularly important for accurate staining of predictive markers (eg, ER/PR, HER2/*neu*) since the interpretation is dependent on the degree of immunoreactivity observed.[19-21] Several studies have described methods for producing standardized, routinely processed pellets of cells lines containing tumors with known quantities of antigen for this purpose.[22-24] For routine quality control, the use of a multi-tissue control block is recommended for this purpose. Several methods have been described, including the "sausage" technique with modifications and, more recently, the use of tissue microarrays, as prepared by automated instruments.[25-29]

Internal positive controls refer to antigens present in the normal tissue structures of the patient tissue being tested. Staining of these structures represents the single best evidence that the antigen has been adequately demonstrated in that tissue section. Documentation by the pathologist that the internal positive controls are appropriately stained is an essential quality assurance measure (see "Interpretation"). Unfortunately, internal positive controls are not always present (eg, ALK-1 protein, herpes virus). Thus, while it is theoretically possible for a laboratory to avoid using a separate positive control tissue for ubiquitous antigens (eg, vascular markers), this will not work for all antigens. Given the antigen density differences described above, exclusive use of internal positive controls does not represent optimal practice. If, however, a laboratory chooses to employ this method, the antigens for which internal controls are used exclusively must be carefully documented in the procedure manual.

Negative tissue controls

The negative tissue control is one or more tissues known to lack the target antigen. The intent of this control is to exclude nonspecific staining by the primary antibody due to improper antibody concentration or, most commonly, to unmasking of unwanted antigens by excessive antigen retrieval. Ideally, the negative tissue controls should be fixed and processed identically to the patient tissue and, like the positive tissue controls, undergo the same antigen retrieval and immunostaining protocol. For laboratories in which it is technically feasible, combining positive and negative tissue controls in a single block using the "sausage" technique or a tissue array is an efficient practice.

Negative tissue controls should assess nonspecific staining in general as well as the specificity of the primary antibody in its direct differential diagnostic application. Examples of the former would include tissues rich in biotin, such as kidney and liver, and keratin and collagen-rich tissues (eg, skin) that tend to bind antibodies nonspecifically. Controls that will assess the degree of endogenous biotin staining are particularly important when employing vigorous antigen retrieval techniques (that tend to unmask endogenous biotin) and a detection method based on biotin labeling (eg, ABC systems).

Examples of negative controls that assess specificity in the differential diagnosis include leiomyoma, which should not stain, in the evaluation of CD117 performance, and the inclusion of a pulmonary adenocarcinoma in negative control blocks for some mesothelioma-associated antigens. Multi-tissue blocks can be prepared that provide simultaneous positive and negative controls for antithetical antigens (eg, kappa/lambda, CD3/CD20, keratin, CD45, and HMB-45).

A separate negative control tissue section may not be needed when testing patient tissues that lack the target antigen, that is, tissues that contain an internal negative control. For example, when assessing a CD20 stain for B cells, the absence of staining in normal T lymphocytes, sinus histiocytes, and lymph node stroma would suggest adequate antibody specificity. While this evaluation is an important quality assurance measure and ensures that the antibody has performed appropriately on that particular tissue section, in most cases it does not provide the same information as a separate multi-tissue negative control due to limited amounts and range of nontarget tissue present. If negative internal controls are routinely used as the only method for negative tissue control, the structures to be evaluated for each antibody and the applicable antibodies should be carefully defined in the procedure manual.

Negative reagent controls

A negative reagent control is used to assess the extent of nonspecific staining in the patient tissue. This control is a separate section of patient tissue that undergoes all aspects of the staining protocol, including slide drying, antigen retrieval, and blocking steps exactly in parallel to the other patient tissue slides except that primary antibody is not applied. A negative reagent control section should be run for each block of patient tissue being stained. In the place of primary antibody this tissue section(s) should ideally receive an antibody of the same species (mouse for monoclonal antibodies, rabbit for polyclonal) and isotype (IgG1, IgG2, IgM) at approximately the same protein concentration. This could be a commercially prepared non-immune serum, marketed for this purpose, or an unrelated antibody. Use of a buffer solution or a non-immune protein solution is considered less than optimal as these do not control for potential nonspecific binding of the detection kit reagents to antibodies.

When an antibody panel includes both polyclonal and monoclonal antibodies, there must be a separate control for each detection system employed unless the secondary reagent is a cocktail that addresses both. As there may be several different antigen retrieval techniques employed, it is reasonable to use a single negative reagent control section that has undergone the most vigorous of the retrieval techniques (eg, enzyme plus steam heat/EDTA buffer). It is possible to use slides in an antibody panel as reciprocal negative controls; however, the circumstances in which this technique can be employed must be carefully delineated in the procedure manual.

Interpretation

A number of published studies, including those summarizing the findings in the College of American Pathologists Immunohistochemistry Survey (MK Program) (see "External quality assessments"), document significant interobserver variability in the interpretation of immunohistochemical stains.[13,15,30-31] This emphasizes the need for careful and precise stain evaluation as an essential element of quality assurance in immunohistochemistry. The pathologist must be aware of the potential interpretative pitfalls including sources of false-positive and false-negative results. Adherence to a set of simple rules, as outlined below, will minimize misinterpretation.

Rule 1. Always review the positive and negative control tissues (or review documentation that they have been reviewed by another pathologist and accepted) for each antibody. Focus particular attention on the tissues expected to be negative to ensure the absence of nonspecific staining.

Rule 2. Carefully review the negative reagent control that accompanies the case (ie, the section of patient tissue that did not receive a primary antibody). There should be no staining. The negative section, if properly prepared, will identify nonspecific staining due to endogenous biotin, which may manifest as a diffuse or granular cytoplasmic stain in epithelial cells. Additionally, review of this section will identify endogenous pigments (eg, melanin, lipofuschin, hemosiderin) that could be misinterpreted as focal positivity.

Rule 3. Attempt to interpret each stain only in areas of well-preserved tissue. Tissue that has dried out at the edge or has been subjected to electrocautery will stain nonspecifically, as will areas of underprocessed tissue (typically in the center of a large tissue block) and necrosis or autolysis.

Rule 4. If the stain appears positive, consider the expected pattern of immunoreactivity.[32] For example, monoclonal antibodies to carcinoembryonic antigen and other carbohydrate-like epitopes typically produce a heterogeneous pattern of cytoplasmic and membranous staining that varies from cell to cell. S100 protein and calretinin should produce both nuclear and cytoplasmic staining. Many antigens (TdT, thyroid transcription factor-1, ER, p53) are exclusively nuclear. Leukocyte antigens (eg, CD20, CD45) should be membranous. Examples of antibody staining patterns can be found in Exhibit 8-2. If the expected pattern is not identified, the result should be regarded as equivocal. In contrast, nonspecific staining due to endogenous proteins in the tissue, endogenous biotin, or overstaining will be typically diffuse, and possibly intense, throughout the tumor, lacking cell-to-cell variability.

Rule 5. Always question a negative result in the absence of an internal positive control. For example, an estrogen receptor negative tumor should be verified whenever possible by the presence of staining in adjacent non-neoplastic ductal epithelium. If there are no expected internal positive controls (eg, p53) or if there is no non-neoplastic tissue in the specimen, repeating the stain on another block may be advisable, particularly if the negative result is unexpected. Appropriate internal controls for a series of common antibodies are summarized in Exhibit 8-2.

Rule 6. Regard with caution any unexpected result when comparing antithetical and associated antigens. A large cell malignant neoplasm, for example, should not be positive for both keratin and leukocyte common antigen. A suspected mesothelioma should not stain for both CEA and calretinin. While aberrant antigen expression does occur, unexpected patterns of immunoreactivity are much more commonly the result of incorrect staining. Similarly, be wary of uncommon patterns, such as estrogen receptor negative, progesterone receptor positive breast cancer. This pattern should occur in less than 5% of cases but is quite common when ER immunoreactivity has been lost due to inadequate tissue fixation and processing. Unexpected results should be confirmed by repeat staining. The repeat should be performed on a different block if tissue preservation is a possible cause. This essential quality assurance process implies the routine use of an antibody panel in differential diagnosis. The use of single antibodies to "confirm" the hematoxylin-eosin diagnosis of a specific tumor type can easily lead to misinterpretation.

External quality assessments

The MK Program of the College of American Pathologists provides unstained sections along with a clinical history and specifications as to which stains should be performed. The laboratory records both stain results and a favored diagnostic interpretation based on history, the histologic appearance, and the immunophenotype. The summary report returned to the laboratory includes the interpretation of the referees as well as statistics on the responses of participants, stratified by antibody preparation used. These materials provide an excellent mechanism of external quality assurance and a source of published benchmarks for reproducibility.[13,30,33] This program also can be used as an intradepartmental mechanism of competency assessment when the slides are reviewed and interpretations recorded individually by all pathologists in the department.

Programs using single sections of a tissue microarray have also been instituted for this purpose. These surveys focus on predictive markers (eg, ER, CD20, c-kit, EGFR, HER-2/*neu*) with the intent of benchmarking and validating laboratory performance.

HistoQIP, a joint program of the College of American Pathologists and the National Society for Histotechnology, offers an assessment of slide staining quality. In contrast to the MK Program, the laboratory is asked to submit a designated stain using tissue processed in that laboratory and the routine laboratory staining protocol. These slides, which currently include two hematoxylin-eosin stains, two special stains, and one immunohistochemical stain per challenge, are reviewed by experienced graders, both histotechnologists and pathologists, using standardized grading criteria. The quality score can be benchmarked against other laboratories in the program using frequency distribution data. Educational materials are also provided, including troubleshooting techniques and photomicrographs of optimal stains.

The United Kingdom National External Quality Assessment Service (UK NEQAS) is available to laboratories outside the United Kingdom and provides a rigorous assessment of slides submitted by participating laboratories as well as staining of sections provided by NEQAS, including comments of the reviewers. Reviews of each antigen assessed, including frequency charts of scores achieved, photomicrographs, and technical information, are published quarterly in the *Journal of Cellular Pathology*, which each participant receives as a member benefit. These reviews have occasionally been published in other journals and provide useful benchmarking data.[12,14,18] Additionally, each laboratory receives an end of year performance record.

Postanalytical phase

Reporting

Guidelines for the incorporation of immunostaining data in anatomic pathology reports,[34] a summary of recommendations from The Council of the Association of Directors of Anatomic and Surgical Pathology, were published in 1992 and include: (1) all immunostaining data should be reported, regardless of perceived significance to the diagnosis; (2) a differential diagnosis justifying the immunostains employed should be provided in the report; and (3) the report should include the nature of the specimen studied (paraffin section, etc), the immunoreagents used (including the clone designation if that potentially impacts the interpretation), and the results of all stains, including all information pertinent to the interpretation (eg, intensity, extent, and subcellular distribution of staining). The Council also strongly emphasized the need to link the immunohistochemistry report, if separate, to the primary pathology report, and to ensure that the results are incorporated into the final diagnosis.

Although it is generally accepted that the technical aspects of the immunostaining protocol need not be reproduced in every report, reporting of predictive markers, such as estrogen and progesterone receptors, Ki-67 proliferation index, and HER2/*neu*, may be a special circumstance. Because the technical aspects can impact the ability of a pathologist at one institution to interpret the results obtained elsewhere and to compare them with published studies, it may be useful to include the primary antibody clone used, the general aspects of the procedure (ie, form of antigen retrieval, detection and amplification methods employed), the criteria or cutoff used to determine a positive result, and either the scoring system employed or, in the case of quantitative evaluations, the method of quantitation (cell counts, image analysis, etc). The report may also include some form of validation, either an independent clinical assessment or a link to a published study using similar methodology.

Although most antibodies used in the clinical laboratory are approved by the Food and Drug Administration (FDA) for in vitro diagnostic use and therefore are not subject to the FDA requirement for a disclaimer, predictive markers are often analyte-specific reagents, subject to this requirement.[35,36] The approved disclaimer with modifications recommended by the College of American Pathologists is presented in Exhibit 8-3.

Quality assurance monitors

Repeat slides

An inadequate immunohistochemical stain may be the result of less than optimal tissue selection and/or processing, antibody failure, or technical factors. It is important for the laboratory to document all requests for repeat stains, the reason for the request, the corrective action performed, and the final outcome. Interaction of the pathologist and technologist on a case-by-case basis is essential for successful troubleshooting. Table 8-2 provides examples of common problems and possible immediate corrective action. More extensive discussions of less than optimal staining and troubleshooting can be found in standard textbooks of immunohistochemistry.[3,4] A useful form for

Table 8-2. Examples of common problems

Reason for Repeat	+/- Tissue Controls	Corrective Action
High background	Adequate	Repeat using different block
High background	High background	Repeat at serial dilutions
Staining only at periphery	Adequate	Repeat using different block or increase antigen retrieval
No/weak staining	Adequate	Repeat using different block
No/weak staining	Weak staining	Repeat using new vial or dilution of primary antibody
Tissue detachment	Adequate	Repeat, increase slide drying

documenting repeat stains is provided in Exhibit 8-4. In a larger laboratory, in which requests are received from multiple pathologists, this information should be aggregated and reviewed frequently by the senior technologist and medical director in order to assess trends and provide more definitive corrective action. Tracking of the actual number of repeats as a percentage of overall slides produced is also a useful long-term quality assurance monitor.

Turnaround time

Immunohistochemistry may add significantly to the overall turnaround time of a surgical pathology or cytopathology case. As these may be high-profile cases, objective monitoring of turnaround time, either periodically through a retrospective audit or prospectively through the routine use of time stamps, is a useful quality assurance measure. Laboratories may choose to separately monitor the time the order was received to slide release and the time required for interpretation and reporting. Exhibit 8-5 provides a simple template for tracking turnaround time.

Audits of pathology reports

A retrospective review of reports from cases utilizing immunohistochemical stains may provide very useful information on the efficacy and efficiency of ordering practices by the pathologists as a group and individually. More importantly, review by a pathologist not involved in the case can provide useful feedback regarding the clarity and completeness of reporting. For each stain performed, the reviewing pathologist should be able to ascertain: (1) the reason that antibody was ordered (ie, the contribution to the differential diagnosis); (2) the result and staining pattern, if appropriate; and (3) whether that antibody contributed materially to the final diagnosis. It may be useful to assess at this time the turnaround time and the presence or absence of an analyte specific reagent (ASR) disclaimer, if appropriate.

Exhibit 8-1. Antibody lot-to-lot comparison

Antibody: _____

Current Lot: _____

Dilution: _____

New Lot: _____

Dilution: _____

Results: _____

_____

Comments: _____

_____

_____

Approved By: _____

Date: _____

Exhibit 8-2. Antibody staining patterns and controls

Stain	Pattern	Tissue Controls	Internal Controls
Actin, smooth muscle	C	Leiomyoma/leiomyosarcoma Sclerosing adenosis, breast	Vascular smooth muscle Myoepithelial cells
Bcl-2	C, M	Follicular hyperplasia Follicular lymphoma	T lymphocytes
Calretinin	N, C	Mesothelioma	Mesothelial cells
CD15	M, Golgi	Hodgkin lymphoma Adenocarcinoma	Granulocytes
CD30	M, Golgi	Hodgkin lymphoma Anaplastic large cell lymphoma Embryonal carcinoma	Plasma cells Immunoblasts
CD31	C	Kaposi sarcoma Breast/colon CA with angiogenesis	Normal endothelium
CD34	C, M	Gastrointestinal stromal tumor Bone marrow with AML Solitary fibrous tumor	Normal endothelium
CD45	M	Non-Hodgkin lymphoma	Lymphocytes
CD56	M	Neuroendocrine CA	Nerves
CD117	C, M	Gastrointestinal stromal tumor Bone marrow with AML Seminoma	Mast cells Interstitial cells, gut
CD138	M	Plasmacytoma	Plasma cells
CEA	C	Colon CA	Granulocytes (Poly)
Chromogranin	C (granular)	Pancreatic endocrine tumor Carcinoid	Mucosal endocrine cells
Desmin	C	Leiomyoma/leiomyosarcoma	Vascular smooth muscle
EMA	C, M	Breast CA	Plasma cells, Glandular epithelium

C: cytoplasmic; M: membranous; N: nuclear

Stain	Pattern	Tissue Controls	Internal Controls
Estrogen/Progesterone Receptors	N	Breast CA, Leiomyosarcoma	Breast, cervical epithelium Myometrium
GFAP	C	Glioblastoma	Normal glial cells
HMB-45	C	Melanoma	Junctional melanocytes
Inhibin	C	Granulosa cell tumor Adrenal cortical adenoma	Ovarian cortex
Kappa	C	Myeloma, kappa monotypic	Plasma cells
Keratin, High Mol Wt (34BE12, CK 5/6)	C	Prostate with adenocarcinoma Squamous carcinoma	Prostatic basal cells
Keratins 7, 20	C	AdenoCA of breast, lung, colon Stomach/bile duct, ovary	Glandular epithelium
p53	N	Serous CA, ovary	None
p63	N	Squamous CA Prostate CA	Myoepithelium Prostatic basal cells
PLAP	M	Seminoma	None
PSA	C	Prostate CA, high grade	Prostate glandular cells
S-100 protein	N, C	Melanoma, Schwannoma	Nerves, Melanocytes
Synaptophysin	C (granular)	Pancreatic endocrine tumor Carcinoid	Mucosal endocrine cells
TdT	N	Thymoma Lymphoblastic lymphoma	Thymic lymphocytes
TTF-1	N	Lung adenocarcinoma	Alveolar lining cells

C: cytoplasmic; M: membranous; N: nuclear

Exhibit 8-3. Analyte specific reagent disclaimer

One or more of the tests in this panel were developed and their performance characteristics determined by Community Hospital Laboratory. They have not been cleared or approved by the US Food and Drug Administration. The FDA has determined that such clearance or approval is not necessary. These tests are used for clinical purposes. They should not be regarded as investigational or for research. This laboratory is regulated under the Clinical Laboratory Improvement Amendments of 1988 (CLIA) as qualified to perform high complexity clinical testing.

Exhibit 8-4. Repeat stains

Repeat Immunohistochemical Stains

Date	Case #	Stain	Reason for Repeat	Corrective Action	Repeat Acceptable?

Exhibit 8-5. Turnaround time

Turnaround Time – Immunohistochemistry

Case #	Date & Time Ordered	Stain / Ordered	Date & Time Initial Slides Released	Repeat or Additional Stains Requested	Date & Time Additional Slides Released	Date Case Verified

References

1. *Quality Assurance for Immunocytochemistry.* Approved Guideline Wayne, PA: NCCLS; 1999. Document MM4-A.

2. Taylor CR. The total test approach to standardization in immunohistochemistry. *Arch Pathol Lab Med.* 2000;124:945-951.

3. Taylor CR, Shi S-R, Barr NJ, Wu N. Techniques of immunohistochemistry: principles, pitfalls, and standardization. In: Dabbs DJ. *Diagnostic Immunohistochemistry.* Philadelphia, Pa: Churchill Livingstone; 2002.

4. Elias JM. *Immunohistopathology: A Practical Approach to Diagnosis.* 2nd ed. Chicago, Ill: ASCP Press; 2003.

5. Chan JKC. Advances in immunohistochemistry: impact on surgical pathology practice. *Semin Diagn Pathol.* 2000;17:170-177.

6. O'Leary TJ. Standardization in immunohistochemistry. *Appl Immunohistochem Mol Morphol.* 2001;9:3-8.

7. Taylor CR. Quality assurance and standardization in immunohistochemistry: a proposal for the annual meeting of the Biological Stain Commission. *Biotech Histochem.* 1992;67:110-117.

8. Shi S-R, Cote RJ, Taylor CR. Antigen retrieval immunohistochemistry: past, present, and future. *J Histochem Cytochem.* 1997;45:327-343.

9. Werner M, Cho HA, Fabiano A, Battifora H. Effect of formalin fixation and processing on immunohistochemistry. *Am J Surg Pathol.* 2000;24:1016-1019.

10. Abbondanzo SL, Allred DC, Lampkin S, et al. Enhancement of immunoreactivity among lymphoid malignant neoplasms in paraffin-embedded tissues by refixation in zinc sulfate-formalin. *Arch Pathol Lab Med.* 1991;115:31-33.

11. Tubbs RR, Bauer TW. Automation of immunohistology. *Arch Pathol Lab Med.* 1989;113:653-657.

12. Rhodes A, Jasani B, Balaton AJ, Miller KD. Immunohistochemical demonstration of oestrogen and progesterone receptors: correlation of standards achieved on in house tumors with that achieved in external quality assurance material in over 150 laboratories from 26 countries. *J Clin Pathol.* 2000;53:292-301.

13. Nagle RB, Tubbs RR, Roche PC, et al. Clinical laboratory assays for HER-2/neu amplification and over expression: quality assurance, standardization, and proficiency testing. *Arch Pathol Lab Med.* 2002;126:803-808.

14. Rhodes A, Jasani B, Balaton AJ, et al. Study of interlaboratory reliability and reproducibility of estrogen and progesterone receptor assays in Europe: documentation of poor reliability and identification of insufficient microwave antigen retrieval time as a major contributory element of unreliable assays. *Am J Clin Pathol.* 2001;115:44-58.

15. Von Wasielewski R, Mengel M, Wiese B, Rudiger T, Muller-Hermelink HK, Kreipe H. Tissue array technology for testing intralaboratory and interobserver reproducibility of immunohistochemical estrogen receptor analysis in a large multicenter trial. *Am J Clin Pathol.* 2002;188:675-682.

16. Hsi ED. A practical approach for evaluating new antibodies in the clinical immunohistochemistry laboratory. *Arch Pathol Lab Med.* 2001;125:289-294.

17. Maxwell P, McCluggage WG. Audit and internal quality control in immunohistochemistry. *J Clin Pathol.* 2000;53:929-932.

18. Varma M, Berney DM, Jasani B, Rhodes A. Technical variations in prostate immunohistochemistry: need for standardization and stringent quality assurance in PSA and PSAP immunostaining. *J Clin Pathol.* 2004;57:687-690.

19. Leake R, Barnes D, Pinder S, et al. Immunohistochemical detection of steroid receptors in breast cancer: a working protocol. *J Clin Pathol.* 2000;53:634-635.

20. Jacobs TW, Gown AM, Yaziji H, et al. HER-2/neu protein expression in breast cancer evaluated by immunohistochemistry: a study of interlaboratory agreement. *Am J Clin Pathol.* 2000;113:251-258.

21. Ellis IO, Bartlett J, Dowsett M, et al. Updated recommendations for HER2 testing in the UK. *J Clin Pathol.* 2004;57:233-237.

22. Riera J, Simpson JF, Tamayo R, et al. Use of cultured cells as a control for quantitative immunocytochemical analysis of estrogen receptor in breast cancer: the Quicgel method. *Am J Clin Pathol.* 1999:111:329-335.

23. Rhodes A, Jasani B, Couturier J, et al. A formalin-fixed, paraffin-processed cell line standard for quality control of immunohistochemical assay of HER-2/neu expression in breast cancer. *Am J Clin Pathol.* 2002;117:81-89.

24. Wick MR, Swanson PE. Targeted controls in immunohistochemistry: a useful approach to quality assurance [editorial]. *Am J Clin Pathol.* 2002;117:7-8.

25. Battifora H, Mehta P. The checkerboard tissue block: an improved multi-tissue control block. *Lab Invest.* 1990;63:722-724.

26. Miller RT. Multi-tumor "sandwich" blocks in immunohistochemistry: simplified method of preparation and practical uses. *Appl Immunohistochem.* 1993;1:156-159.

27. Weirauch M. Multitissue control block for immunohistochemistry. *Lab Med.* 1999; 30:448-449.

28. Hsu FD, Nielsen TO, Alkushi A, et al. Tissue microarrays are an effective quality assurance tool for diagnostic immunohistochemistry. *Mod Pathol.* 2002;15:1374-1380.

29. Packeisen J, Buerger H, Krech R, Boecker W. Tissue microarrays: a new approach for quality control in immunohistochemistry. *J Clin Pathol.* 2002;55:613-615.

30. Wold LE, Corwin DJ, Rickert RR, Pettigrew N, Tubbs RR. Interlaboratory variability of immunohistochemical stains: results of the Cell Markers Survey of the College of American Pathologists. *Arch Pathol Lab Med.* 1989;113:680-683.

31. Rudiger T, Hofler H, Kreipe H-H, et al. Quality assurance in immunohistochemistry: results of an interlaboratory trial involving 172 pathologists. *Am J Surg Pathol.* 2002;26:873-882.

32. Cheuk W, Chan JKC. Subcellular localization of immunohistochemical signals: knowledge of the ultrastructural or biologic features of the antigens helps predict the signal localization and proper interpretation of immunostains. *Int J Surg Pathol.* 2004;12:185-206.

33. Tubbs RR, Nagle R, Leslie K, et al. Extension of useful reagent shelf life beyond manufacturers' recommendations. *Arch Pathol Lab Med.* 1998; 122:1051-1052.

34. Banks PM. Incorporation of immunostaining data in anatomic pathology reports. *Am J Surg Pathol.* 1992;16:808-810.

35. Taylor CR. FDA issues final rule for classification and reclassification of immunohistochemistry reagents and kits. *Am J Clin Pathol.* 1999;111:443-444.

36. Swanson PE. Labels, disclaimers and rules (oh, my!): analyte-specific reagents and practice of immunohistochemistry. *Am J Clin Pathol.* 1999;111:445-448.

Quality management in cytopathology

Theresa M. Voytek, MD
Dina R. Mody, MD
Diane D. Davey, MD

Introduction

This chapter is directed toward cytopathology quality assurance (QA) and continuous quality improvement (CQI), rather than routine quality control (QC) activities, but some QA/QC activities, especially in gynecological cytology, require continuous monitoring and are mandated by the Clinical Laboratory Improvement Amendments of 1988 (CLIA '88) regulations. Other areas are more appropriate for focused periodic monitors and will vary depending on the practice environment. The following sections will differentiate required from suggested monitors. Specific areas selected for monitors should be reviewed at least annually to assess effectiveness and changing patterns of practice.

Laboratories should consistently document review activities and monitor their effectiveness in improving performance. Even though many of the gynecological cytology monitors have been mandated for continuous review, laboratories should still try to evaluate and document their effectiveness.

Cytology laboratories vary greatly in size, staffing, and scope of practice. While this manual offers general guidelines and examples, each laboratory should design a program that meets its needs and conforms to appropriate regulatory and accreditation standards. For example, hospital-based laboratories must follow the increasingly rigorous requirements of the Joint Commission on Accreditation of Healthcare Organizations (JCAHO) regarding the delineation of clinical privileges and peer review activities. Large laboratories may use hierarchical review programs extensively and also benefit from extensive databases, which are useful for developing internal standards of practice and quantifying quality review activities. The small laboratory and the solo practitioner face unique challenges in attempting to establish quality assurance programs. Regular continuing educational experiences, cytohistologic correlation, liberal use of external consultation, and participation in interlaboratory comparison programs are useful quality assurance tools for all laboratories, especially in those smaller settings.

At the end of the chapter, a collection of tables is provided to assist in the documentation of these monitors. These are provided only as examples and are not required; nor are all the monitors present in the tables required. Alternatively, laboratories may generate and store similar data in computer systems or develop other tables more suitable for the particular laboratory setting. Regardless of the method used, periodic review of monitors with documentation is required.

Definitions

Current terminology for evaluating cytological performance is variable, and national standards do not yet exist. Internal consistency in the use of terminology for quality assurance activities is critical. The following definitions are offered as guidelines for data analysis.

Discrepant interpretation. An interpretation in which two different opinions on the same specimen, or on different but related specimens, would impact a patient management decision. This may occur if there is a difference in diagnosis between the cytological specimen and subsequent histological specimen, or between two individuals reviewing the same specimen. This applies to both exfoliative and aspiration cytology. A more specific definition of discrepant interpretation used commonly in gynecologic cytology is a two-step difference in diagnosis between the cytology and subsequent histology. A Pap interpretation of low-grade squamous intraepithelial lesion (LSIL) in which the biopsy shows carcinoma, and a Pap test reported as high-grade squamous intraepithelial lesion (HSIL), with concurrent biopsy showing only benign squamous metaplasia, are examples of two-step discrepancies. Lesser variations in diagnosis are useful to consider and review primarily for educational purposes.

False-negative specimen. A negative result from a patient who has disease. In gynecological cytology, a false-negative specimen is one in which the cytological specimen is negative for intraepithelial lesion or malignancy, but subsequent follow-up reveals an abnormality (SIL or carcinoma). False-negative specimens may be due to sampling, interpretive, or screening problems, and are often useful to categorize.

False-positive specimen. A positive result from a patient without disease. In gynecological cytology, a false-positive specimen is one in which the cytological specimen is interpreted as abnormal (SIL or carcinoma), but the subsequent follow-up/biopsy shows no malignancy or epithelial lesion.

Sensitivity. The ability of a test (eg, Pap test) to identify correctly the presence of a lesion or malignancy. Sensitivity may be further categorized as screening/interpretive sensitivity or sampling sensitivity. Sensitivity = (True-Positive / [True-Positive + False-Negative]) x 100.

Specificity. The ability of a test (eg, Pap test) to identify correctly the absence of a lesion or malignancy. Specificity = (True-Negative / [True-Negative + False-Positive]) x 100.

Hierarchical review. The sequential review of the same specimen by individuals with increasing levels of experience and responsibility.

Peer review. Sequential review of the same specimen by individuals who have similar levels of responsibility and experience.

Concurrent review. Review of the same specimen by at least two individuals prior to reporting the interpretation.

Retrospective review. Review and correlation of the original interpretation with subsequent information from cytological, histological, or clinical studies.

Benchmarking. Comparison of the laboratory's performance with that of other laboratories (eg, College of American Pathologists [CAP] interlaboratory comparison programs).

Quality assurance in cytopathology and CLIA '88

Historical overview

The most dramatic changes in quality assurance practices have resulted from the Clinical Laboratory Improvement Amendments of 1988 (CLIA '88). Prior to 1967, the practice of cytopathology in the United States was virtually unregulated. The Clinical Laboratory Improvement Act of 1967 (CLIA '67) established the first federally mandated policies for quality control in cytopathology, including personnel standards, retention of slides, 10% rescreening of benign gynecological specimens, and review of suspicious or abnormal smears by the director or supervisor. In 1987, articles in the lay press and television documentaries appeared about high false-negative rates in Pap test interpretations, poor performance in some cytopathology laboratories, and excessive cytotechnologist workloads. In 1988, the Centers for Disease Control and Prevention (CDC) sponsored two meetings on quality assurance in cytopathology, and congressional hearings were held to explore problems in clinical laboratories.[1,2] Prompted by this media attention, congressional testimony, and data from the CDC conferences and other sources, Congress passed CLIA '88. The final regulations were implemented in September of 1992, with the exception of proficiency testing, which was made effective in 2005.[3-5]

CLIA '88 and accreditation monitors

In each of the following sections, the quality assurance regulations and monitors mandated by CLIA '88 are indicated by italic text. In some areas, the specific sections of CLIA '88 regulations are given. The CAP Laboratory Accreditation Program (LAP) checklist requirements are commonly similar or identical to CLIA '88 regulations and are continually updated. When there are LAP as well as JCAHO requirements that are not part of CLIA, these are generally specified in the text. Note that not all LAP checklist items and CLIA '88 requirements for laboratories are detailed in this manual since the aim is QA/CQI activities; readers are also referred to these documents.

General cytology laboratory procedures

All laboratory procedures should be thoroughly documented in a procedure manual. The laboratory director must review procedure manuals annually, and laboratories should document that analysts are knowledgeable about the contents (relevant to the scope of their activities). The following subjects that are included in general cytology laboratory procedures contain mandated monitors.

Specimen acceptance and adequacy

Written instructions for collection and submission of specimens should be available to physicians and clinics, including types of fixatives to be used. Transportation of specimens to the laboratory should also be evaluated and monitored.

Each laboratory should have written criteria for rejecting specimens [CLIA '88 493.1242(a)(7)]. These criteria may include unlabeled slides or specimens, broken slides, or specimens without requisitions. The specimen (slide or container) should be directly labeled. *The requisition should include patient name (and/or unique identifier), sex, specimen source, pertinent clinical information, requesting physician's or other authorized person's name, and date of specimen collection. For gynecological specimens, the date of last menstrual period should be included as well as age or date of birth and pertinent history of previous abnormal reports, treatment, or biopsy [CLIA '88 493.1241(a-e)].* The LAP checklist also requires date of birth or age for all specimens. A gross description of the specimen (number of slides received, quantity and appearance of fluid specimens) should be included with accessioning/processing procedures.

Gynecological specimen adequacy is discussed below (see "Gynecological cytology quality assurance"). For most non-gynecological specimens, certain cell types should be present in sufficient numbers to be considered adequate for evaluation. For example, sputum specimens should contain alveolar macrophages. Washings and lavage of certain body sites (bladder, bronchoalveolar) should contain at least minimal numbers of cells representative of those sites. In contrast, normal cerebrospinal fluids have very few cells, so scantly cellular spinal fluid should not be labeled as unsatisfactory. For fine-needle aspiration (FNA) biopsy specimens, it is critical not to label unsatisfactory or nondiagnostic specimens as "negative" (see "Fine-needle aspiration cytology"). A distinction should be made between specimens rejected prior to processing and those that are rejected after processing and review (unsatisfactory or inadequate for evaluation).

Suggested monitors

Log of rejected/unsatisfactory specimens (see Table 9-1). This log should include the submitting clinician or location as well as specimen type and reasons for rejection. Clinicians should be notified of rejected/unsatisfactory specimens. If the log shows an increased incidence (percent unsatisfactory) from a certain physician or location, education on submission should occur and be documented.

Specimen preparation and staining

For gynecological specimens, a Papanicolaou (or modified) stain must be used [CLIA '88 493.1274(b)(1)]. A Papanicolaou or permanent nuclear stain should be used in non-gynecological specimens. A Wright-Giemsa stain or modification (eg, Diff-Quik® and others) may be useful for assessing aspirate specimens and some fluid specimens. Coverslips should adequately cover the material. Liquid coverslips are not satisfactory. The quality of the preparations and stains should be monitored daily by a supervisory technologist or lab director (LAP checklist requirement). A general Cytopathology Problem Log may also be useful to identify and track a variety of laboratory problems and trends that could negatively impact the laboratory's quality (see Table 9-2). When special stains for organisms or cell products are used, appropriate control slides should also be reviewed.

There should be measures in place to prevent cross-contamination between samples [CLIA '88 493.1274(b)(2)]. Laboratories should document these measures in their procedure manuals. The greatest potential for cross-contamination occurs when staining very cellular non-gynecologic specimens. Although gynecologic cases have less potential for cross-contamination and may be stained in batches, they should be stained separately from non-gynecologic specimens. Laboratories may develop their own methods to prevent cross-contamination of specimens. Several possible methods include:

- Use a rapid stain, such as toluidine blue, to detect cellular cases. Filter all stains after each cellular specimen is stained.
- Use a staining sequence, staining paucicellular specimens before highly cellular ones, filtering or changing solutions after staining a cellular specimen. For example, stain clear cerebrospinal fluids first, followed by more cellular specimens such as direct smears from sediment of highly cellular specimens (ie, highly cellular, positive body fluids).
- Use at least two sets of stains, and while using one, filter the other so that a clean set is always available.
- Document each time the stains are filtered or changed. This will keep track of these steps to prevent cross-contamination as well as provide documentation during laboratory inspections.

Occasionally, possible cross-contamination is identified despite precautionary measures. The specimens with possible contaminants should be compared with other positive cases stained that day. Repeat preparations may be useful in some cases. The laboratory should document how the case(s) has been resolved.

Suggested monitors

Log of quality control staining procedures (see Tables 9-3 and 9-4). This can include the date and number of times the stains are filtered and changed, a record of stain evaluation for quality (clarity of cells and smear background), and any problems noted and their resolution. If an automatic stainer is used, the timing should be checked and recorded on a regular basis, and the machine should be serviced according to the manufacturer's specifications.

Workload monitors in cytology

The laboratory must maintain records of the workload of individual cytotechnologists and screening pathologists, and workload limits must not be exceeded [CLIA '88 493.1257(b)].

Individuals who manually screen cytological preparations may examine no more than 100 slides per day (24-hour period) in no less than 8 hours [CLIA '88 493.1274(d)(2)]. This limit includes gynecological and non-gynecological specimens as well as quality control rescreens. Laboratories must also comply with state regulations. Some states have a maximum workload limit lower than 100. Most slides will count as one slide. Non-gynecologic slides using a liquid-based preparation technique in which the cell dispersion occupies one-half or less of the slide are the exception and may count as one-half slide (examples include cytospin®, monolayer or liquid-based preparations, and filters). All gynecologic slides, both conventional and liquid-based preparations, count as whole slides. Slides should be screened over an 8-hour day; those individuals working part time or performing other duties must prorate their slide limit. The laboratory is responsible for keeping records that document the number of slides screened and the number of hours devoted to screening.

The laboratory director/technical supervisor must establish workload limits for each individual based on capabilities and performance using evaluations of 10% negative QC rescreens and cytotechnologist-pathologist interpretation correlation data [CLIA '88 493.1274(d)(1)]. Evidence of review must be documented at least every 6 months. The 100-slide limit is an absolute maximum and must not be used as a production goal. Laboratories with numerous complex specimens or less experienced personnel may choose to set lower limits. Additional factors, such as laboratory and cytotechnologist statistics, CAP Interlaboratory Comparison Program in Cervicovaginal Cytology (PAP Program) performance, and previous workload records, may be useful to consider in setting and reviewing workload limits. The maximum daily workload limit for cytotechnologists using computer-assisted screening devices may be higher than 100; however, care should be taken to set reasonable maximum workload limits based upon the individual ability of the cytotechnologist to avoid compromising screening accuracy.

Required monitors

Logs of slides screened per individual per day may be kept manually or generated by computer (see Table 9-5). A second monitor should record workload limits for each individual screener, with documentation of review every six months by the laboratory director. The laboratory director should use negative quality-control rescreens and cytotechnologist-cytopathologist correlation data to determine the workload limit Other factors that can be considered include cytotechnologist statistics compared with laboratory statistics, performance on proficiency tests or interlaboratory comparison programs, and competency assessment. Comparison of cytotechnologist abnormal rate (pickup rate) and unsatisfactory rate to the laboratory average rate is very useful to evaluate cytotechnologists' screening performance. For example, if a cytotechnologist's abnormal rate is well below the laboratory average, it may indicate a screening problem. The director should then investigate further by evaluating other quality monitors. Rescreening of additional negative cases screened by the cytotechnologist during the period reflected by the statistic may also be indicated. Based upon the evaluation, the director may decide to lower the workload limit (see Tables 9-6 through 9-9).

The laboratory should have written policies and procedures for employee competency assessment [CLIA '88 493.1235]. Although cytotechnologist competency assessment is a primary focus of this chapter, laboratories should also assess and monitor the competency of other personnel. Table 9-10 shows an example of cytopreparatory competency assessment.

Personnel standards

Recent regulations specify qualifications standards for the laboratory director (technical supervisor) and cytotechnologists [CLIA '88 493.1449, 493.1469, 493.1483]. The LAP checklist is similar.

Cytopathology reports and records

CLIA '88, JCAHO, and/or the CAP LAP checklist require certain report/record components. *CLIA '88 requires records which document unique patient and specimen identification, the date and time of specimen receipt into the laboratory, the condition and disposition of specimens that do not meet the laboratory's criteria for specimen acceptability, the dates of testing, and the identity of personnel who performed the tests [CLIA '88 493.1283 and 493.1291].*

The report must give the laboratory name and address, and the test result (including disposition of unsatisfactory specimens). Reports must be retained at least 10 years. The date of reporting is required by JCAHO. The LAP checklist requires the following components:

- Name of patient
- Date of birth and/or age
- Unique patient number
- Attending physician and/or clinic
- Dates of collection, receipt, and reporting of specimen
- Source of cytological material
- Cytology accession number
- Laboratory names and addresses
- Description of specimen on receipt (including unacceptable specimens and gross description)
- Test performed, including imaging device used, if applicable
- Interpretation (result of examination)
- Comments and recommendations, when appropriate
- Pathologist's signature, when appropriate

Documentation of oral communication may be included in the report or in laboratory records. *If corrected reports are issued, the basis of the correction must be indicated [CLIA '88 493.1257(f)].* The report distribution, internal review of reports, and mechanisms for handling complaints can be undertaken in the same manner as for surgical pathology.

Laboratory records must identify those who have reviewed the slides. For cases requiring cytopathologist evaluation, the report should indicate the pathologist's name, initials, or signature in written or electronic form. The reviewing pathologist's name should be distinct from other names on the report (eg, laboratory director). *The electronic signature should be authorized and released by the pathologist who performed the review [CLIA '88 493.1274(e)(2)].*

Gynecological cytology quality assurance

The following divisions of this section include mandated CLIA monitors:

- Specimen acceptance and adequacy
- Screening and reporting of gynecological specimens
- Rescreening of negative cases
- Cytological/histological correlation and clinical follow-up
- Retrospective reviews
- Measures of quality of screening/interpretive performance
- Descriptive statistics of interpretations

All of these have components mandated by CLIA '88, with regulations effective September 1, 1992, and most are also included in the LAP and/or JCAHO checklists. The LAP checklist also requires records of consultations. Proficiency testing was implemented in 2005. All individuals who examine gynecological preparations (cytotechnologists and pathologists) must participate in a CMS-approved proficiency testing program in gynecologic cytopathology. The approved Clinical and Laboratory Standards Institute (formerly NCCLS) guideline for the Papanicolaou technique is a useful reference for gynecological specimen collection and Papanicolaou staining.[6] In addition, the American Society of Cytopathology has published cervical cytology practice guidelines.[7]

Specimen acceptance and adequacy

The laboratory report must clearly distinguish specimens that are unsatisfactory for diagnostic interpretation [CLIA '88 493.1274(e)(4)]. The Bethesda System, in its updated 2001 version,[8] recognizes the importance of adequacy in the evaluation of the specimen and subdivides this examination into two categories:

1. Satisfactory for evaluation: describe presence or absence of endocervical/ transformation zone component and any other quality indicators
2. Unsatisfactory for evaluation (specify reason)

Laboratory criteria for adequacy should be documented in the procedure manual. A satisfactory specimen is appropriately labeled, is accompanied by relevant patient information, is technically acceptable, and contains adequate numbers of well-preserved and visualized squamous cells. The presence or absence of a transformation zone component should be described in specimens from women with a cervix. At least 10 well-preserved endocervical or squamous metaplastic cells should be observed to report that a transformation zone component is present. When there is partial or complete atrophy, it may be difficult to determine the presence of a transformation zone component. Parabasal cells should not be counted as transformation zone components, and laboratories may include commentary about the difficulty of identifying a transformation zone component in these cases. Bethesda 2001 recommended that the intermediate "Satisfactory but limited by ..." category be eliminated. However, partially obscuring factors (50% to 75% of cells obscured by blood, inflammation, or other) should still be mentioned following the satisfactory designation. Laboratories may also add educational comments concerning the significance of the transformation zone component, other quality indicators, and the importance of regular screening.

Unsatisfactory specimens should include wording to designate whether the specimen was rejected or fully evaluated in order to document laboratory work performed. The suggested wording is:

- Specimen rejected ... (specify reason)
- Specimen processed and examined, but unsatisfactory for evaluation of epithelial abnormality because of ... (specify reason)

The first category includes unlabeled specimens and those slides broken beyond repair, and would not be considered eligible for Medicare billing. The second category includes specimens with marked obscuring factors (more than 75% of cells obscured) as well as those with insufficient squamous cells. It is important to identify unsatisfactory specimens, as studies have shown that women with unsatisfactory Paps (especially those with obscuring factors) may have a higher likelihood of SIL or malignancy on follow-up specimens.[9] Bethesda 2001 suggested criteria for minimum squamous cellularity. An adequate conventional Pap should have an estimated minimum of approximately 8000 to 12,000 well-preserved/visualized squamous cells. Individual cells should not be counted, and reference images are provided to help estimate cellularity. Liquid-based Paps should have a minimum of 5000 well-preserved/visualized squamous cells, and tables providing average cell number per microscopic field are available. Cellularity may be difficult to estimate in some cases with cytolysis, atrophy, and cell clustering, and strict objective criteria may not be applicable to every case. Hierarchical review is recommended in borderline cases. Laboratories should also consider factors such as clinical history, previous abnormalities, hormonal status and presence of transformation zone elements. The squamous cellularity criteria were developed for use with cervical cytology specimens. Laboratories should exercise judgment in evaluating cellularity of vaginal specimens based on clinical and screening history.

Caveat: Any abnormal cell is significant regardless of specimen adequacy.
The specimen containing abnormal cells must never be classified as unsatisfactory.
CLIA '88 requires the laboratory to ensure that diagnostic interpretations are not reported on unsatisfactory smears. Similarly, the specimen with malignant cells can never be classified as other than satisfactory. Additionally, any clinically suspicious lesion must undergo biopsy irrespective of cytological findings.

Required monitor

Volume of unsatisfactory specimens.

Suggested monitors

It is useful to identify submitting clinicians or clinics so that appropriate education can occur if an excess incidence of unsatisfactory specimens occurs. Also, some intralaboratory (peer or hierarchical) review of unsatisfactory specimens should take place to achieve some uniformity in application of adequacy criteria. The supervisor or pathologist may choose to sign out all unsatisfactory Paps and a portion of satisfactory Paps with quality indicators. Monitors of individual rates of specimen adequacy among various cytotechnologists and pathologists may be useful quality improvement parameters. This is especially important as new criteria are adopted in the laboratory. Suggestions (either oral or in the report) or educational comments to clinicians may be useful in certain situations.

Screening and reporting of gynecological specimens

All gynecological slides should be thoroughly screened by a cytotechnologist(s)/pathologist(s) in a certified laboratory [CLIA '88 493.1274 (a)]. All reactive/reparative, atypical, premalignant, and malignant cases must be referred to the pathologist (hierarchical review) for final interpretation [CLIA '88 493.1274 (e)(1)]. Documentation should be maintained (see Table 9-6). Written records of previous cytological/histological specimens, if available, should be reviewed prior to final reporting.

Narrative descriptive nomenclature must be used in reporting Gynecological specimens [CLIA '88 493.1274(e)(5)]. The numerical classification system is inappropriate. Standard methods of reporting squamous lesions in gynecological cytology include the Bethesda System, Cervical Intraepithelial Neoplasia (CIN), and the degrees of dysplasia. A clear, concise, and descriptive nomenclature is essential to ensure communication between the laboratory and the clinician. A 2003 CAP PAP Program questionnaire showed widespread acceptance of the Bethesda 2001 system (85.5%).[10]

Written educational comments or suggestions for further diagnostic studies are optional but can be useful. The 2003 PAP Program survey showed that 56% of responding laboratories routinely use educational notes in reports. Any recommendations or comments should be consistent with clinical management guidelines (for examples, see reference 11). In addition to the written report, verbal communication may be necessary in cases where further diagnostic studies are indicated. Such communication should be documented, preferably on the report.

Discordant interpretations (between cytotechnologist(s) and pathologist(s), or between two pathologists) should be resolved, if possible, prior to final reporting. Review at a multiheaded microscope with discussion of the case is a useful educational exercise.

Review of abnormal gynecological cases

A second pathologist (internal or external) can perform peer review of abnormal gynecological specimens, ranging from those with atypical squamous cells (ASC) to malignancy. This review can include all cases or a sample, depending on the type of laboratory practice.

Examples: In small laboratories/hospitals with limited gynecological case volumes, the pathologist may elect to review the abnormal cases with a colleague prior to sign-out. If a significant discrepancy in interpretation exists between the cytotechnologist and pathologist, case review with a colleague is recommended prior to final reporting. Similarly, the pathologist may choose to refer a portion of abnormal cases to an external consultant. Indicators for referral would include difficult diagnostic cases and those not encountered routinely in the practice.

In larger settings with high gynecological case volumes, focused review of a subgroup of abnormal cases may be performed. Possible indicators include difficult cases in which an interpretation might affect patient management (eg, reparative versus premalignant and malignant cellular changes; radiation and/or chemotherapy effects on cells; glandular epithelial abnormalities).[12] A review of cases with ASC may aid the pathologists in arriving at a consensus diagnosis. The ratio of ASC to SIL cases may also be a useful monitor to identify possible problems with diagnostic criteria for ASC.[13] This ratio can be compared with those of other laboratories with similar patient populations or to the established ratio of the laboratory.

The interpretation and name or initials of the peer reviewer should be recorded on the report or within the laboratory records. For external consultation, the referring physician should be informed of the reviewer's report, and the original maintained within the laboratory files.

Rescreening of negative cases

Bethesda 2001 recommends reporting negative cases as "Negative for Intraepithelial Lesion and Malignancy." There is no standard that has been scientifically validated specifying the percentage of negative cases that should be rescreened. *CLIA '88 regulations [493.1274(c)(1)] specify that at least*

10% of negative gynecological specimens from each cytotechnologist be rescreened, and that both randomly selected cases and those from "high-risk" individuals (based on available patient information) be included in the rescreened specimens. The review must be performed by an experienced qualified cytotechnologist, supervisor, or pathologist and must be completed prior to reporting. At present, the only exception to this regulation is for slides primarily screened by the Focal Point primary screening system (Tripath). In this process, at least 15% quality control rescreening of the highest scoring "review" slides is required.

Laboratories should determine the number of slides to be rescreened and how these cases are to be selected based on their patient population and on their practice environment. Random rescreening may be a useful tool to determine the laboratory's error rate or false-negative proportion. Review of previously negative specimens when a new high-grade abnormality is detected is an important component of negative case review (see "Retrospective reviews"). Negative specimens in areas considered problematic diagnostically should also be used; examples include marked inflammatory changes, partially obscured cases, and changes due to therapy.

Rescreening negative slides should be an integral part of the evaluation of new technologists. The rescreening process should allow identification of the original cytotechnologist in laboratory records.

Required quality control

Rescreening is required of at least 10% of negative gynecologic cytology cases, including those from high-risk patients. Written documentation should be maintained.

Cytological/histological correlation and clinical follow-up

The laboratory must compare all gynecological cytology reports with an interpretation of HSIL or carcinoma with the histopathology report, if available, in the laboratory (either on site or in storage) and determine the cause of any discrepancies [CLIA '88 493.1274(c)(2)]. Although cytohistologic correlation is mandated by CLIA '88, methods for analysis are not specified. A system-wide approach may result in improved patient care. As the histologic biopsy may not always be the "gold standard," reasons for discrepancy should be pursued. The use of an algorithm can be useful for cytohistologic correlation including non-laboratory factors.[14] The Pap test and the histologic specimen are independently reviewed. The latter should be adequately sectioned and oriented so a continuous lining epithelium including transformation zone is observed. If available, negative cytology cases should also be reviewed whenever the histology is positive. It is important to stress that some agreed-upon definition of diagnostic discrepancy be established (see "Definitions"). Peer review of noncorrelating specimens may be helpful to achieve consensus. Results can be summarized on a regular basis so trends and improvements can be tracked (see Table 9-11).

A CAP Q-Probes study of 22,429 paired cervicovaginal cytology and biopsy specimens revealed a discrepancy rate of 16.5%.[15] The Pap test sensitivity was 89%, specificity 65%, and positive predictive value 89%. The majority of discrepancies were due to cytology and biopsy sampling errors, rather than screening or interpretive errors, and the result of factors outside the control of the laboratory. Of patients with LSIL on cytology, 18% had HSIL on follow-up biopsy. It is therefore unrealistic to expect perfect correlation between cervicovaginal cytology and cervicovaginal biopsy. While cervicovaginal cytology is appropriately regarded as a screening test and colposcopic biopsy the "gold standard" confirmatory test, both tests are subject to sampling error and, in some cases, the Pap test may better represent the cervical pathology than the biopsy. If in the case of a patient with a Pap diagnosis of HSIL and negative biopsy follow-up, the cause of the discrepancy is determined to be a biopsy sampling error and review of the Pap confirms the original interpretation, the clinician may proceed to definitive treatment (ie, LEEP). Therefore Pap-biopsy correlation is critical for appropriate patient management.

Communication of findings with clinicians is vital. If specimens are correlated concurrently, a comment can be included in the pathology report, when appropriate. Direct communication via phone calls or letters is useful to discuss individual patient follow-up. Amended reports may be necessary if screening, interpretive, or technical problems are detected that would affect current patient care. Interdepartmental committees or conferences are another avenue to discuss cytohistologic correlation results.

Histological follow-up may not always be available. In these cases, other follow-up studies such as human papillomavirus (HPV) testing, repeat Pap tests, and colposcopic examination findings may be informative (see Table 9-12). Follow-up is particularly important in cases of HSIL, glandular abnormalities, and carcinoma.

Retrospective reviews

Previously negative cytological and relevant histological material should be reviewed to correlate results whenever current material shows an abnormality that could have been overlooked in the prior specimen.[16,17] *Federal regulations stipulate that negative or normal specimens obtained within the previous 5 years either onsite or in storage be reviewed whenever a high-grade SIL or malignant lesion is first detected [CLIA '88 493.127457 (c)(3)].* This review should be documented. The pathologist should also review any previous cases in which rescreening by the technologist detects possible abnormalities. The laboratory should have established criteria regarding what constitutes a significant variance in the interpretation. It is useful to define a discrepant interpretation as one that affects current patient care. *If significant abnormalities are found on review which would affect current patient care, the clinician must be notified and an amended report issued [CLIA '88 493.1274 (c)(3)].* Although retrospective reviews may not reflect current cytotechnologist competency and should not be a major component in the evaluation of cytotechnologist performance, they are a useful educational tool and can detect screening/interpretive problem areas for the laboratory.

Required monitor

Review of previous negative cytology specimens in cases with new high-grade lesion or carcinoma is a required monitor (see Table 9-13).

Measures of quality of screening/interpretive performance

The laboratory must evaluate individual performance in comparison to overall laboratory performance and document discrepancies and corrective action if appropriate [CLIA '88 493.1274(c)(6)]. Although the regulations do not specify the method of comparison, laboratories are required to use 10% random rescreening data and cytotechnologist/pathologist interpretation correlation data for cytotechnologist workload determination. Other methods that can be used to monitor performance include targeted rescreening, retrospective rescreening, calculation of pickup rates (or percent abnormal specimens), and tracking of cytological/histological correlation data.

These various methods of evaluating screening performance each have advantages and disadvantages, depending on a variety of factors including laboratory size and caseload. Some of the methods may be most useful as education and training devices.

Random rescreening of cases may be a useful method to compare performance in relatively large laboratories (several cytotechnologists and large, evenly distributed gynecologic case volume). This method should use a randomizing strategy to select cases. Some laboratories use this data to calculate an estimated false-negative proportion (FNP). The FNP is the percentage of women with cervical neoplastic or preneoplastic lesions who have a negative Pap test. It is defined as the number of false-negative reports divided by the total number of women with a cervical abnormality (FNP=FN/[TP+FN]), where FN is the number of false-negative reports and TP is the number of true positive cases. Although FNP is a commonly used statistic in quality assessment, it may not accurately reflect the laboratory performance because the false-negative rate of rescreening, which can be substantial, is not taken into account.

Targeted rescreening of high-risk patients has also been discussed and is mandated under CLIA '88. It is very useful as a quality assurance mechanism. Since the population is preselected, rescreening will not be a random sample and numerical error rate calculation is difficult. Some comparison of individual screening abilities may be possible using descriptive terms rather than numerical data.

Comparison of pickup rates between individuals. In this discussion, pickup rate refers to the percentage of abnormal cases diagnosed by an individual; for example, the sum of atypical, premalignant, and positive cases is divided by the total cases examined. This method is useful in most laboratories, providing those individual screeners and/or pathologists view a similar mix of cases. A total pickup rate can be calculated for each individual and compared with the laboratory pickup rate. This type of calculation may be feasible on a quarterly basis. Alternatively, various degrees of abnormalities can be compared for individuals. Since numbers for each category will be smaller than the total abnormal pickup rate, the frequency of performing calculations may be once or twice a year. In addition to calculating pickup rates for squamous abnormalities, it may be useful to compare pickup rates for unsatisfactory Paps and other findings.

Evaluation of interpretive errors and cytohistologic correlation may be useful in comparing interpretive abilities and is very useful for educational purposes. Since it may be difficult to perform statistically valid comparisons, descriptive terms are likely to be useful for most laboratories (see specific sections).

Comparison of cytotechnologist/pathologist correlation. This correlation data should be considered in the determination of cytotechnologist workload limits and can be monitored in a variety of ways left to the discretion of the laboratory. One way to track this data is by assigning diagnostic scores to calculate correlation discrepancy scores. These data can then be summarized in histograms, as follows.

1. Cytologic (or histologic) diagnoses are assigned scores as follows:

Negative	0
Reactive/Repair	1
ASC(US-H)/AGC	1.5
LSIL/CIN I	2
HSIL/CIN II	3
HSIL/CIN III	4
Squamous cell ca	5
Adenocarcinoma	5

2. The score of the pathologist diagnosis is subtracted from the score of the cytotechnologist = discrepancy score.

3. Each case is then given a correlation score by using the following formula:

$$\frac{M-|D|}{M} \times 100$$

where M is the maximum possible score (in the above scoring system), and |D| is the absolute value of the discrepancy score.

For the above scoring system, the formula would read:

$$\frac{5-|D|}{5} \times 100$$

4. The data for a given time period are summarized in a histogram in which each bar represents the number of cases with each discrepancy score. The correlation scores are averaged for the total number of slides and reported as a single number for the same time period.

5. This method of analyzing and presenting cytotechnologist/pathologist discrepancies is optional and, in most cases, requires computer support.

Given the following data, a histogram can be created to provide a visual picture of pathologist/cytotechnologist correlation for a specific time period.

1. In one week, a pathologist reviewed 357 slides previously screened by the cytotechnologist and found discrepancies in 83. In 2 cases, there was a +2.5 discrepancy score; 2 were +1.50; 1 was +1.00; and 41 cases had discrepancy scores of +0.50. Of those cases with negative discrepancy scores, 23 were -0.50; 13 were -1.00; and 1 was -1.50. In the remaining 274 cases, there was no discrepancy (score 0.00).

Number of Cases	Cytotech Score	Pathologist Score	Discrepancy Score	Correlation Score	Total Correlation Score
2	4	1.5	2.5	0.5	1.0
1	1.5	0	1.5	0.7	0.7
1	3	1.5	1.5	0.7	0.7
1	1	0	1.0	0.8	0.8
30	1.5	1	0.5	0.9	27.0
11	2	1.5	0.5	0.9	9.9
274	NA	NA	0.0	1	274.0
15	1	1.5	-0.5	.09	13.5
8	1.5	2	-0.5	.09	7.2
8	0	1	-1.0	0.8	6.4
5	1	2	-1.0	0.8	4.0
1	0	1.5	-1.5	0.7	0.7
357					345.9

Cumulative Correlation Score = 345.9/357x100= **96.6**

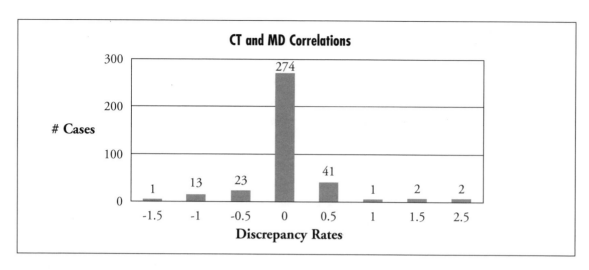

For any of these methods, the laboratory should establish a threshold for performing additional case reviews of individuals falling outside the norm for the laboratory. The thresholds should be set after determining what random variation can be expected, which is not due to variation in performance. This threshold may be continuously refined as the laboratory gains experience with the monitor and can serve to reflect the laboratory's CQI activities. For example, if an individual has a pickup rate more than X% below the lab average or an error rate more than Z% above the lab average, the lab may elect to perform some additional case review. Similarly, if pickup rates for a pathologist are significantly above the lab average, some of the individual's cases (for example, atypia and low-grade lesions) should be reviewed for possible overcalls.

Review of discrepancies between individuals

Individual cytotechnologists and pathologists should receive feedback on cytologic interpretations and cytological/histological correlations. If possible, discrepancies that would affect current patient management should be resolved by the pathologist prior to sign-out of the case. If, during retrospective case reviews, the reviewing pathologist has a significantly different opinion, the original pathologist should be consulted; an amended report should be sent out if the reviewed diagnosis is confirmed and current patient management would be affected. It is also suggested that discrepancies between individual cytotechnologists and pathologists be regularly reviewed for any patterns. Records of discrepancies can be kept manually or in a computer system, and reviewed by the pathologist. If any patterns are detected or thresholds exceeded, the problems should be addressed suitably through the department's quality improvement mechanisms (eg, in-service education, review of cases at a multi-headed microscope). Such cases indicate problem areas in the laboratory and are usually of educational value.

Suggested monitor

Records of discrepancies.

Consultations

Records of internal and external case consultations should be maintained (LAP checklist requirement). The consultant's opinion and name or initials can be recorded separately or within the cytology report.

Review of unknown cases

A number of formal educational and proficiency testing programs provide selected unknown cases that may be reviewed and interpretations compared with those of peers and experts. Some of these programs are sponsored by state agencies and other professional societies or private organizations. Such programs are suitable for quality improvement and continuing education purposes. Examples are listed below:

- The College of American Pathologists Interlaboratory Comparison Program in Cervicovaginal Cytology (PAP Program)
- The American Society for Clinical Pathology (ASCP) and Midwest Institute for Medical Education (MIME) glass slide programs

Records of participation and results of these programs should be maintained within the laboratory. Any controversial or discrepant cases should be reviewed individually or discussed in laboratory meetings. Laboratories should maintain documentation of proficiency testing performance of individuals for at least 2 years.

Descriptive statistics of interpretations

Statistical records are mandated [CLIA '88 493.1257(d)(4)] and include the annual number of cytologic specimens and number processed by specimen type. The volume of cases by interpretation including the number of unsatisfactory cases is required. The annual number of gynecologic specimens where rescreen of a negative or normal results in reclassification as malignant or premalignant also must be documented. Similarly, the number of gynecological cases in which cytology and histology are discrepant and the number of HSIL and malignant gynecologic cases in which histologic follow-up is available are required.

There are several ways in which these descriptive statistics can be summarized. A tabular form may be useful, but a more narrative form also can be used (see Table 9-14).

Turnaround time

Turnaround times for gynecologic cytology vary considerably due to personnel shortages, and national standards have not been established. The turnaround time for gynecological cytology should satisfy the clinical needs of referring physicians, and the laboratory should be responsive to special patient circumstances such as surgical and other therapeutic procedures.

Interlaboratory comparison data

Interlaboratory comparison programs provide laboratories with useful benchmarking data for laboratory processes. The PAP Program consists of unknown glass slide material, as well as questionnaires on current laboratory practices. This program, begun in 1989 with 207 participant laboratories, has served over 1900 laboratories in recent years.[18-20] The CAP Q-Probes program also has included several cytology exercises.[21-24] Laboratories can use data from these programs to establish indicators and thresholds. Indicators are tools used to measure an organization's performance of functions, processes, and outcomes over time. A threshold can be set based on past laboratory performance as well as the benchmark of average or optimal laboratory performance.

Descriptive Pap statistics

The LAP checklist publishes reporting rate distributions for various Pap results. An example of a benchmark indicator is cervicovaginal Pap test adequacy rate. Based on a 2003 questionnaire survey, the median rate of unsatisfactory specimens was 0.5%. The median ASCUS (atypical squamous cells of undetermined significance) rate determined by the survey was 3.1% for conventional Paps and 4.1% for liquid-based preparations. The median ASC/SIL+ ratio was 1.4 for conventional and 1.3 for liquid-based Pap tests. The median reported ASC/SIL+ ratio has decreased since the 1996 CAP survey when it was 2.0. Because ASCUS (ASC) and SIL rates may vary more with practice setting, the ratio ASC/SIL+ may be more useful as a benchmark.[13]

Conventional Laboratory Percentile – Reporting Rate							
Category	5th	10th	25th	50th	75th	90th	95th
ASC-US (%)	0.5	0.9	1.6	3.1	4.8	7.0	9.7
ASC-H (%)	0.0	0.0	0.0	0.1	0.3	1.0	2.1
LSIL (%)	0.3	0.5	0.8	1.4	2.1	4.0	5.6
HSIL+ (%)	0.1	0.1	0.2	0.4	0.7	1.5	2.2
ASC/SIL+(%)	0.5	0.7	1.0	1.4	2.3	3.3	3.7
AGC (%)	0.0	0.0	0.1	0.2	0.5	1.0	1.3
Unsatisfactory (%)	0.0	0.1	0.2	0.5	1.0	2.0	3.1

Liquid-Based Preparations Laboratory Percentile – Reporting Rate							
Category	5th	10th	25th	50th	75th	90th	95th
ASC-US (%)	0.9	1.4	2.6	4.1	5.9	8.9	11.0
ASC-H (%)	0.0	0.0	0.1	0.2	0.4	1.0	1.5
LSIL (%)	0.8	1.1	1.6	2.4	3.6	5.4	6.9
HSIL+ (%)	0.1	0.2	0.4	0.5	0.9	1.6	2.0
ASC/SIL+(%)	0.4	0.6	1.0	1.3	1.9	2.5	3.1
AGC (%)	0.0	0.0	0.1	0.2	0.3	0.7	1.0
Unsatisfactory (%)	0.0	0.0	0.2	0.4	0.8	1.2	1.6

PAP Program

The 2003 PAP Program enrolled 742 laboratories in the conventional PAP Program and 1060 in its liquid-based programs. In 2003, the false-negative rate for conventional validated Paps was 1.5% for laboratories, 1.1% for cytotechnologists, and 2.2% for pathologists. The false-positive rate was 1.5% for laboratories, 1.7% for cytotechnologists, and 2.5% for pathologists. For liquid-based ThinPrep validated slides, the false-negative rate was 1.9% for laboratories, 1.2% for cytotechnologists, and 3.3% for pathologists. The false-positive rate was 1.1% for laboratories, 1.0% for cytotechnologists, and 2.2% for pathologists. However, as these figures only include interpretive/screening discrepancies in cases that were subjected to multiple rescreens and vigorous validation criteria, they are not reflective of and likely underestimate error rates in daily practice settings. The CAP publishes annual PAP Program year-end summary reports for its participants, which contain useful benchmark data for all diagnostic categories used in the program.

Retrospective rescreening

A 1993 Q-Probes study of 338 laboratories found an aggregate false-negative rate of 10.1% when negative prior Paps from patients with current HSIL/cancer were rescreened.[24] The false-negative rate was defined as the ratio of all previous cases with a rescreen diagnosis of SIL or carcinoma divided by the number of all rescreened cases. When very critical retrospective rescreening studies are performed, and when the threshold for "error" is low, the false-negative rate is higher. The aggregate false-negative fraction in the Q-Probes retrospective rescreening study was 20% when cases with atypical squamous or glandular cells on review were included as errors. Higher rates have been reported from academic centers, so an upper acceptable limit cannot be established. Therefore error rates from retrospective rescreening exercises are not directly comparable to those obtained by concurrent random rescreening.[25,26]

Follow-up of women with abnormal Paps

A Q-Probes study of 16,132 cases revealed that follow-up within 1 year was obtained for 86% of patients with a cytologic diagnosis of carcinoma, 87% with HSIL, 83% with LSIL, and 85% with glandular intraepithelial lesion.[22,27] A larger percentage of patients with LSIL received follow-up when a recommendation for follow-up (repeat Pap or colposcopy/biopsy) was included in the cytology report, compared with those whose report did not include a recommendation.

New technologies in gynecologic cytopathology

Although the Pap test is the most successful cancer screening test, and the conventional Pap smear remains a highly effective and inexpensive screening test to prevent cervical cancer, new technologies have been developed in gynecological cytology to further improve the rate of detection of cervical neoplasia by decreasing the false-negative rate. Examples of current technologies that may improve Pap test sensitivity include improved collection methods, cytopreparatory techniques such as liquid-based preparation, automated screening devices, and HPV testing.

Liquid-based Pap tests improve specimen quality by providing immediate fixation, improving cellular sub-sampling, and providing more uniform cell presentation with fewer obscuring factors. Several studies support an increased detection rate of SIL. Due to these differences, laboratories should consider monitoring separate pickup rate and rescreening error rate statistics for conventional and liquid-based methods. Liquid-based specimens also lend themselves to additional testing, particularly for HPV, the causative agent of nearly all cervical SILs and carcinomas. Recent studies have demonstrated HPV testing to be helpful in the management of patients with ASCUS.

A major advantage of this test is that it can be performed on the same sample as the Pap test, avoiding a second patient office visit. Laboratories that perform HPV testing can also use the test as a quality assurance monitor of its atypical squamous cells (ASC) cases. It may be educational to correlate ASC cases with their HPV results.

Automated screening devices may be useful as a primary screening method to select cases requiring further review and a minority of negative cases to be reported without manual screening. Computer-assisted screening devices may allow increased productivity by selecting the fields most likely to contain abnormal cells for the cytotechnologist to evaluate, without requiring full manual screening unless an abnormality is detected in these fields.

There should be documentation of adherence to the manufacturers' recommended protocols for implementation of new instrumentation in the laboratory. Laboratories should demonstrate performance specifications comparable to those established by the manufacturer [CLIA 493.1253]. There should be documentation of ongoing instrument maintenance and function checks for all devices as defined by the manufacturer [CLIA 493.1254]. Included are slide preparation and screening devices. If there are no manufacturer's recommendations for validation and instrument monitoring, the laboratory must specify the validation procedure used and document system monitoring.

While the Food and Drug Administration is responsible for approval of new devices, the laboratory director is responsible for assessing the feasibility of new technologies for the laboratory. Laboratory practices may vary based upon a variety of factors, including patient characteristics, laboratory size/case volume, and cost. The director is also responsible for implementation of new technologies and ensuring the competency of cytopathology staff. Whatever methods used, a new method's sensitivity should equal or exceed conventional methodology without a significant loss of specificity, and the results should be reproducible. Performance in detection of high-grade lesions and cancers is considered most critical. The method should also detect unsatisfactory cases. The standard of practice is determined over time by the cytopathology profession.[28,29]

Liability issues/risk management in gynecologic cytopathology

Quality assurance and continuous quality improvement programs are instrumental in ensuring a high standard of patient care. Laboratories must also comply with cytology accrediting agencies and governmental regulations. Despite tremendous efforts to improve the accuracy and sensitivity of the Pap test, false-negative tests still occur. Although the limitations of the Pap test are well known to most cytopathologists, they are less well understood by clinicians and virtually unknown to most patients. The limitations of the Pap test should be communicated to physicians and their patients to prevent unrealistic expectations of the test.[30]

Much information about the Pap test can be communicated via the Pap report. The report can include a comment about the limitations of the Pap test and suggestions for patient follow-up. The report should contain a statement about specimen adequacy. It is important to communicate that the Pap test is a screening test, rather than a diagnosis. In accordance with Bethesda 2001, laboratories may choose to report the Pap test as an "interpretation" or "result," rather than a "diagnosis." A comment indicating that the Pap test has a significant false-negative rate, and that a negative test does not exclude the presence of an abnormality, helps to educate patients and encourages scheduling of regular Pap tests.

Suggestions on Pap reports may also ensure appropriate patient management. A CAP Q-Probes study of 16,312 cases revealed that the type of recommendation significantly influenced the type of follow-up, for example, repeat Pap versus biopsy.[22]

The American Society of Colposcopy and Cervical Pathology (ASCCP) met in September 2001 and established evidence-based practice guidelines for the management of cervical lesions. Suggestions provided in the Pap report for patient management should be consistent with these guidelines.[11]

Unfortunately, practice at a high standard of care does not eliminate the potential for litigation. Because the outcome of cases brought to litigation is often determined by the testimony of expert pathologist witnesses who have reviewed the cytologic slides, guidelines have been developed in an effort to ensure fairness of this process.

In the case of litigation, the case should be reviewed with specific guidelines to most accurately assess whether negligence has occurred. The slide(s) should be reviewed by an individual with significant experience in cytopathology, without knowledge of the clinical outcome, in an environment that is similar to a normal practice environment. The expert should review the original slide(s) with the same clinical information that was available to the original pathologist. The standard of care should be that of a reasonable and prudent practitioner, and the finding of a false-negative test is not necessarily evidence of practice below this standard. The witness should receive compensation that reflects only the time and effort expended on the case; compensation should not be contingent upon the outcome of the case.[31,32]

Laboratories should have policies to protect the integrity of current slides. Some laboratories have a policy of not sending out negative slides for review. A request for a negative slide is often to obtain information for litigation rather than for patient management, and it is recommended that the laboratory consult with a risk manager before releasing negative slides. Pap test slides can be discarded after 5 years.

Non-gynecological cytology quality assurance

Several indicators for non-gynecologic specimens can be monitored. Indicators may include:

- Peer review (prospective or retrospective, intra- or extradepartmental)*
- Site-specific review — retrospective review of a specific organ or specimen type
- Cytology/histology correlation and follow-up*
- Laboratory statistics*,**
- Cytotechnologist/cytopathologist correlation
- Turnaround time*
- Continuing medical education and benchmarking tools*

    *   CAP LAP
    ** CLIA '88

Sign-out and review of non-gynecological cases

All non-gynecological specimens must be reviewed by a pathologist (hierarchical review), and this should be stated in the procedure manual [CLIA '88 493.1274(e)(3)]. The report must be signed (written or electronically) by the pathologist who performed the review.

If records of previous pertinent histological/cytological specimens are available, these should be reviewed prior to signing out the current case. Cytotechnologists should receive feedback on performance and case diagnoses (see "Review of discrepancies between individuals" in the "Gynecological cytology" section).

Descriptive statistics

General statistical records should include the number of non-gynecological cytology specimens and diagnostic categories, including those unsatisfactory for evaluation. Other statistics may vary, but could include the types/sources of specimens and the collection technique (eg, FNA of lung, sputum). Laboratories also may find it useful to monitor numbers of positive/suspicious cases continuously or for limited periods. Statistical comparison of non-gynecological diagnoses by individuals is not performed given the small numbers and varied sources of specimens encountered in most laboratories.

Suggested monitor

See Table 9-14 for a sample method of tabulating statistics.

Peer review

Prospective review of abnormal non-gynecological cases

In difficult areas of non-gynecological cytology, where definitive therapy may be based on a positive cytology result, concurrent peer review of positive, suspicious, or atypical cases may be useful. FNAs, respiratory brushings and washings, or fluid specimens are examples of specimen types for which prospective peer review may be useful. For example, two pathologists could review every new diagnosis of malignancy. Significant discrepancies in diagnoses that would affect patient care (between cytotechnologist and pathologist, or between two pathologists) should be resolved, if possible, prior to sign-out. Group review and discussion is a useful tool that helps maintain consistency in laboratory diagnosis.

Examples: Small practices with few non-gynecological specimens may choose to refer cases for general quality assurance for outside consultation.[33] Such cases could include malignant cases without histologic confirmation, unusual cases, or organ-specific specimens (eg, breast FNA, cerebrospinal fluid, thyroid FNA). In larger practices, concurrent review may be integrated into daily cytology practice.

Another useful mechanism is to define experts within the group for various organ or specimen types and to refer problem cases to such "internal experts." In some laboratories, there is a scheduled quality assurance pathologist; in other settings, an informal consultation is used.

Retrospective review of non-gynecological specimens (including negatives)

For gynecological specimens, there is educational value in reviewing previous negative cervicovaginal specimens when a significant abnormality is found in a current specimen or in a cervical biopsy. The value of such retrospective reviews of negative non-gynecological specimens is not well established. Sampling procedures and skill of procurer vary significantly, and therefore many (if not most) of the possible "false-negative" results are due to sampling rather than screening or interpretive problems. Laboratories will probably find such retrospective reviews to be most useful if a certain specimen type is analyzed over a specified time period as a focused monitor (see "Site-specific review" below)

Another form of retrospective peer review is a random review of a fixed number of cases on a weekly or monthly basis. Each laboratory should determine the number or percentage of cases and the review format. These should be done in a timely manner such that if a significant discrepancy that would affect patient care is found, the physician is notified as soon as possible.

Site-specific review/focused review

Retrospective review of an organ or site over a specific time frame can be helpful. This type of review can be correlated with histologic follow-up, peer review, turnaround times, laboratory statistics, etc. This review may identify means to improve sampling and/or processing methods, as well as monitoring screening and/or interpretation problems.

Example: Laboratory personnel note that very few bladder washing specimens yield clinically useful information, while many corresponding bladder biopsies show urothelial carcinoma or a dysplastic process. This area of practice is selected for a focused study in which all bladder washings for the past year are correlated with the results of bladder biopsies taken within the same time period. On review, only 30% of the cases with documented pathology have an abnormal cytologic result (atypical, suspicious, or positive). Reviews of many of the cytologically negative cases with positive histology show scant cellularity. The pathologist discusses the findings with staff urologists, who institute changes to specimen collection. Follow-up studies 6 months later show a higher sensitivity of bladder washings for neoplastic processes.

Cytology/histology correlation and follow-up

Some documented effort to obtain histologic correlation in abnormal or positive non-gynecological specimens is required in the LAP program.

The CAP Cytopathology Committee recommends that laboratories correlate positive and suspicious cytologic specimens with concurrent histologic biopsies, when available. For some non-gynecological specimens, the cytology material may be the first positive or suspicious material obtained in that patient. In such cases, it is suggested that follow-up histologic material or clinical information be sought. Examples are brushing specimens (respiratory, gastrointestinal), many fine-needle aspiration specimens, and any controversial specimens. This may be either a continuous monitor or focused audit. In other cases, the patient may have a known history of malignancy, and no future histologic biopsies are expected. Examples are positive body fluids from patients with previously diagnosed malignancies. In these cases, previous histological or cytological material should be pulled and reviewed along with the current cytological material if there is any question as to the interpretation.

Histological follow-up may not always be available. Other types of clinical follow-up may be useful in these circumstances, including letters to the clinician, selected chart reviews, serum tumor marker studies, and radiological studies. When an infectious organism is detected (respiratory specimens, etc), follow-up cultures may be of educational value.

Suggested monitors

A small laboratory may choose to continually monitor all positive or suspicious cases for histological/clinical follow-up. A large lab may perform a focused monitor of a certain specimen type. In either case, files are searched for histological/other follow-up after a certain time period has elapsed. If discrepant diagnoses are found, the slides of both cytology and histology should be pulled for review, with comments made as to whether the discrepancy represents a sampling, screening, or interpretive error. Table 9-15 is an example of a useful format for documentation.

As a CQI mechanism, significant screening/interpretive errors may be discussed at cytology education or quality improvement meetings (see "Retrospective review of non-gynecological specimens").

Turnaround time

Turnaround time for non-gynecological specimens should be monitored. Because results are important for immediate patient care decisions, turnaround time for non-gynecologic specimens should be of the same order as for surgical biopsies. Although few studies address the subject for non-gynecologic cytology specimens, the authors of a recent CAP Q-Probes study recommend a turnaround time of 2 working days for most routine cases.[34] The CAP LAP Cytopathology Checklist requires that 90% of routine non-gynecologic cases be signed out within 2 working days. Cases requiring additional studies, such as immunocytochemistry or molecular studies, may take longer. Longer reporting times may also be allowed for screening (as opposed to diagnostic) specimens, such as screening urine specimens. The laboratory may identify specific specimen or patient types for which longer turnaround time is clinically acceptable. These exceptions should be listed in the policy manual.

Suggested monitor

Review turnaround time for a period of time. A clerk or secretary should identify reports on non-gynecological specimens and record days elapsed between the day the specimen was received and the day the specimen was signed out. Median days and ranges can then be calculated. If the median is longer than the threshold, reasons for long turnaround time can be investigated and possible corrective action instituted.

Continuing education and benchmarking

Continuing medical education for pathologists and cytotechnologists in non-gynecological cytology is an integral part of quality improvement. This may include journal subscriptions, internal conferences (such as microscopic consensus conferences, lecture review, or interactive sign-out), participation in mailed education programs such as the CAP Interlaboratory Comparison Program for Non-Gynecologic Cytopathology (NGC Program), ASCP Check Samples or related programs from MIME, teleconferences, and cytology courses and meetings.

Fine-needle aspiration cytology quality assurance

Fine-needle aspiration cytology (FNA) is a specialized area of cytopathology. Quality assurance includes all elements reviewed previously, but since FNA may be a definitive diagnostic procedure and the pathologist may be involved with obtaining the specimen, additional elements must be considered. These include (1) informed consent, (2) specimen procurement, (3) specimen adequacy, (4) interpretation by a pathologist knowledgeable in this technique, and (5) communication with the clinicians involved with the procedure.[35]

Informed consent

Informed consent is generally required to perform invasive procedures. A consent form for FNA should be developed and periodically reviewed. Specific items that should be included in the document include:

- Patient name
- Physician(s) performing the procedure
- Biopsy site
- Patient's signature and date

- Statement of patient's assent that the procedure, along with its risks and benefits, has been explained either verbally or through a descriptive brochure
- Statement of patient's assent that he/she is satisfied and that he/she has received sufficient information necessary to make an informed decision regarding the procedure

The consent form may include statements regarding:

- Anesthesia
- Signature of witness(es)
- Disclaimer on diagnostic accuracy
- Accuracy of the procedure (medical literature, institution or individual physician experience)
- Explanation to include information on false-negative and false-positive interpretations and possible complications

In some institutions or practices, an informed consent form may not be needed, provided the procedure and its complications and expectations are explained to the patient and there is documentation to that effect.[36]

Periodic review of consent forms for completeness of information and presence of appropriate signatures is a suggested monitor.

Specimen procurement

The FNA may be performed by the pathologist, treating physician, or radiologist. Appropriate utilization of this technique is directly dependent on the expertise of the physician performing the procedure. The facilities should be adequate for examination and proper positioning of the patient. There should be adequate working space for preparing the slides, and if microscopic assessment for specimen adequacy is performed, a microscope and quick cytology staining set-up is necessary. Supplies should be available for culturing aspirated material when clinically indicated. As in most patient care areas, there should be access to resuscitative equipment and available personnel to perform cardiopulmonary resuscitation. Follow-up mechanisms to detect complications of the procedure may be useful.

Specimen adequacy

Guidelines should be developed to determine the adequacy of the specimen. Possible ways to ensure adequacy in most specimens include: (1) gross visual assessment of cellular material aspirated when smears are prepared; (2) immediate microscopic assessment of adequacy using a quick cytology stain prior to releasing the patient; and (3) multiple needle aspirations. The specific method used will depend on individual circumstances and the ease of repeating the procedure if the first specimen is nondiagnostic.[37-42]

Guidelines for interpretation

A pathologist who is familiar with the diagnostic criteria of FNA should interpret the specimen. A definitive diagnosis should only be made when adequate numbers of well-preserved cells are present and clinical history is available. Documented concurrent peer review of problematic cases is suggested. If circumstances permit, peer review of all positive aspirates may be useful, particularly when definitive therapy is planned or the technique/site is new to the laboratory.

Report

All reports and oral communication, when indicated, should be relayed to the appropriate clinician in the same manner as a histological biopsy. There should be clear written communication between the pathologist and the referring physician. Oral communication should be documented. Reports optimally should include a reference to the adequacy of the specimen and/or its limitation. The report and diagnosis should distinguish those specimens that have adequate material and do not show a malignant process, those specimens that are inadequate, and those specimens that are nondiagnostic. Recommendations for further studies may be appropriate in the report.

Correlation studies

Clinical or histologic follow-up correlation studies are an important aspect of FNA quality assurance. This is especially critical when a laboratory has little prior experience with this technique. Correlation of all FNA sites may be performed periodically, or a specific organ site may be selected for a focused audit.[43] Small laboratories or laboratories new to this technique may aim for follow-up on all aspirates. Larger or experienced laboratories benefit from focused organ-site audits.

Example: As a focused monitor, all breast aspirates from the prior year are correlated with histology. Documentation of cytological results may be recorded (Table 9-15).

The histological follow-up (positive, benign, other, no follow-up) is charted. If no histological follow-up is found for the positive and suspicious results, the patient chart is reviewed or the clinician is contacted. Slides from cases with discrepancies are pulled and reviewed with documentation. In this example, cytology slides from benign and unsatisfactory FNAs, but positive histology, should be reviewed. Similarly, any cases with suspicious or positive cytology, but benign follow-up, should also be reviewed. Discrepancies can be categorized as sampling error or interpretation error. Sensitivity can be calculated by adding the positive and suspicious aspirates, and dividing this sum by the total number of patients with satisfactory aspirates and positive histology. Numbers of false-positive and suspicious aspirates (specificity problems) can also be tallied.

If sensitivity is low due to sampling error, an attempt should be made to improve specimen adequacy over the next several months. If there is a problem with interpretive errors, false-positive or false-suspicious results, additional continuing education or peer review mechanisms should be instituted. If it is determined that some patients do not receive appropriate follow-up biopsies or other clinical studies, the clinicians should be contacted and educated. If significant problems in communication exist, appropriate changes in reporting mechanisms should be made.

The same organ site can then be studied again several months after changes have been implemented to ensure that improvement has occurred.

Index of tables

Table 9-1. Cytopathology rejected specimen log

Date	Patient Name/ID#	Clinician	Specimen Type	Reason Rejected	Notification/ Resolution

Table 9-2. Cytopathology problem log
Examples include lost specimen, client complaint, laboratory error, amended report, and prolonged TAT.

Date	Problem	Recommendation/ Action	Follow-up/ Resolution

Table 9-3. Cytopathology stain quality evaluation

Date	QC Tech	Gyn Stain				Non-Gyn Stain			
		Case #	Sat Y/N	Problem	Resolution	Case #	Sat Y/N	Problem	Resolution

Table 9-4. Cytopathology stain maintenance

Stain/Reagent	Date Filtered	Date Changed	Staff

Table 9-5. Cytotechnologist daily slide totals

Cytotechnologist:					
Date	Gyn Primary Screens	Gyn Rescreens	Non-Gyn Slides	Total Slides	Total Hours Screened

Table 9-6. Daily cytotechnologist interpretation log

Cytotechnologist:

Date	Case #	ADEQ	NEG	NEG (Refer to Path)	Reactive/ Repair	ORG	ASC	AGC	LSIL	HSIL	CA	

Table 9-7. Monthly cytotechnologist gyn statistics

Cytotechnologist:

Year:

	Jan #/%	Feb #/%	Mar #/%	Apr #/%	May #/%	Jun #/%	Jul #/%	Aug #/%	Sept #/%	Oct #/%	Nov #/%	Dec #/%
UNSAT												
NEG												
NEG*												
ORG												
ASC-US												
ASC-H												
AGC												
LSIL												
HSIL												
CA												
TOTAL ABNL												
ASC/ SIL+												

*Negative cases referred to the pathologist   ASC= Atypical Squamous Cells   AGC = Atypical Glandular cells   LSIL= Low Grade Squamous Intraepithelial lesion   HSIL= High Grade Squamous Intraepithelial lesion   CA= Cancer   ABNL= Abnormal   ORG = Organism

Table 9-8. Cytotechnologist workload assessment

CYTOTECHNOLOGIST_____

NEGATIVE RESCREENS

Total Rescreened slides _____   Date: _____ to _____

Summary of discrepancies:

                              CYTOTECHNOLOGIST   LAB AVERAGE

Unsat rate:

Organisms missed:

Epithelial abnormalities:

INTERPRETIVE DISCREPANCIES: Date: _____to _____

                              CYTOTECHNOLOGIST   LAB AVERAGE

Discrepancy rate:

STATISTICAL COMPARISONS (PICK-UP RATES): Date: _____to _____

                              CYTOTECHNOLOGIST   LAB AVERAGE

    % Unsat:

    % Negative:

    % Abnormal:

    ASC/SIL+:

Maximum workload limit for period _____ has been set at

_____ slides per hour = _____ slides per day.

Date _____

Cytotechnologist _____   Technical Supervisor _____

Table 9-9. Cytotechnologist competency assessment

CYTOTECHNOLOGIST_____

SATISFACTORY   NEEDS IMPROVEMENT

1. Rescreen Discrepancies

2. Gyn Statistics

3. Pathologist/Cytotech Discrepancies

4. Non-Gyn Screening

5. Final Report and Billing Accuracy

6. PAP Program

7. FNA Adequacy Assessments

8. Knowledge of Procedure
   Manual Contents

9. Other

Comments:

_____

_____

_____

_____

_____

_____

_____

_____

_____   _____   _____
Cytotechnologist   Supervisor   Date

Table 9-10. Cytopreparatory personnel competency assessment

STAFF MEMBER _____

	SATISFACTORY	NEEDS IMPROVEMENT

1. Specimen Identification/Acceptance

2. Accessioning/Labeling/Computer Entry

3. Slide Preparation
   (all methods performed)

4. Staining (all used in lab)

5. Coverslipping

6. Knowledge of Procedures in Manuals

7. Other

Comments:

_____

_____

_____

_____

_____

_____

_____

_____

_____

_____   _____   _____
Employee   Supervisor   Date

Table 9-11. Gyn cytology/histology correlation log

Cyto Case #	Original Interpretation	Reviewer Interpretation	Biopsy Case # & Interpretation	Reviewer Interpretation	Discrepancy Type*	Comments/ Resolution

* Discrepancy Type:

0=None, A=Cytology Sampling, B=Colposcopic Sampling, C=Histology Technical, D=Histology Interp, E=Cytology Interp, F=Cytology Screening, G=Other, H=Combined

Table 9-12. Cytology follow-up correlations

Case #	Specimen Type	Cytologic Interpretation	Follow-up Histology	Follow-up Other*	Comment

* i.e., HPV testing, repeat Pap test, colposcopic examination

Table 9-13. Cytopathology 5-year retrospective reviews

(For New Cases of HSIL and CA)

Date: _____

Reviewer: _____

Current Case # / Interpretation: _____

Previous Negative Case #	Previous Interpretation	+/- Discrepant Interpretation*	Comment/ Action

* Discrepancy that would affect current patient care (current interpretation)

Table 9-14. Cytopathology statistics: gyn and non-gyn

Date: _____ to _____

	CONVENTIONAL	LIQUID-BASED
TOTAL CYTOLOGY CASES	_____	_____
GYNECOLOGIC CASES	_____	_____
Unsat	_____	_____
Negative	_____	_____
ASC-US	_____	_____
ASC-H	_____	_____
AGC	_____	_____
LSIL	_____	_____
HSIL	_____	_____
CA	_____	_____
ASC(US-H)/SIL+	_____	_____
GYN TAT	_____	_____
GYN QC DISCREPANCIES:		
Organisms	_____	_____
Adequacy	_____	_____
Epithelial	_____	_____
CYTOLOGY/HISTOLOGY DISCREPANCIES:	_____	
# OF HSIL+ WITH HISTOLOGY FOLLOW-UP:	_____	
RECLASSIFIED AS PREMALIG. OR MALIG. ON RESCREEN:	_____	
GYN TAT:	_____	
TOTAL NON-GYN CASES:	_____	
FNAs:	_____	
SUSPICIOUS OR POSITIVE:	_____	
CYTO/HISTO DISCREPANCIES:	_____	
NON-GYN TAT:	_____	
AMENDED REPORTS:	_____	
CONSULTATIONS:	_____	

Table 9-15. Focused cytologic/histologic correlation

Specimen Type: _____
Date: _____ to _____

Cyto Case #	Diagnosis	Biopsy Case #	Diagnosis	Correlation Y/N	Discrepancy Type	Action

NEG – Negative/Benign
SUSP – Suspicious
POS – Positive
OTH – Other
UNSAT – Unsatisfactory

CSE – Cytology sampling error
CIE – Cytology interpretive/screening error
BSE – Biopsy sampling error
BIE – Biopsy interpretive error
NFU – No follow-up

Table 9-16. Cytopathology quality improvement plan

Cytopathology Quality Improvement Plan for the Year _____

Department of Pathology
XYZ

The goal of the Quality Management Plan is to provide a means of monitoring the accuracy and completeness of diagnostic reporting by members of _____ cytology staff and to identify potential areas for improvement. Results of monitoring will be reported at _____ meetings and information provided to the participant pathologists and cytotechnologists on a quarterly basis or as deemed necessary. In addition, variant reports identified in the monitoring processes are communicated via _____ (by whom and to whom). Components of the plan for the year _____ include the following:

A. Monthly monitoring of quality management indicators:
- Cytopathologist to cytotechnologist correlation (gyn only)
- Cytology-histology correlation
- Turnaround time (non-gyn only)
- Statistics (gyn and non-gyn)
- Peer Review (prospective)

B. Quarterly monitoring of quality management indicators
- Cytopathologist peer review (intradepartmental and extradepartmental – retrospective)

C. Site-specific reviews (semi-annual or annual if indicated)

D. Cytotechnologist Evaluation and Workload Limits (every 6 months)

E. Continuous mechanisms of quality improvement
- HSIL/Carcinoma look back (gyn only)
- Incomplete requisition/Missing clinical information (gyn and non-gyn)

F. External audit mechanisms
- CAP – Interlaboratory Comparison Program in Gynecologic Cytopathology
- CAP – Interlaboratory Comparison Program in Non-Gynecologic Cytopathology

The results of all monitors are summarized in annual reports with emphasis on identifying trends and target areas for improvement. Areas of concern are reviewed by _____ at (what time) _____ in order to formulate strategies for improvement. Monitors will be modified or added depending upon the potential for identifying new areas for improvement.

Director of Pathology

References

1. Paris AL. Conference on the state of the art in quality control measures for diagnostic cytology laboratories. *Acta Cytol.* 1989;33:423-426.

2. Solomon D. Introduction to the proceedings of the conference on the state of the art in quality control measures for diagnostic cytology laboratories. *Acta Cytol.* 1989;33:427-430.

3. Triol JL, Goodell RM. *ASCT Cytopathology Quality Assurance Guide.* Raleigh, NC: American Society for Cytotechnology; 2001.

4. Clinical Laboratory Improvement Amendments of 1988. Final Rule. *Fed Reg.* 1992;57:7001-7186. Current CLIA regulations (including all changes through 01/24/2003) available at: http://www.phppo.cdc.gov/clia/regs/toc.aspx. Accessed March 3, 2005.

5. Forum: Legislation and regulations governing the field of cytology: review and update. In: Schmidt WA, ed. *Cytopathology Annual.* Baltimore, Md: Williams & Wilkins; 1992:197-253.

6. *Papanicolaou Technique. Approved Guideline.* 2nd ed. Wayne, Pa: NCCLS; 2001. Document GP15-A2.

7. American Society of Cytopathology. Cervical Cytology Practice Guidelines. *Acta Cytol.* 2001;45:201-226.

8. Solomon D, Nayar R, eds. *The Bethesda System for Reporting Cervical Cytology.* 2nd ed. New York: Springer-Verlag; 2004.

9. Ransdell JS, Davey DD, Zaleski S. Clinicopathologic correlation of the unsatisfactory Papanicolaou smear. *Cancer.* 1997;81:139-143.

10. Davey DD, Neal MH, Wilbur DC, Colgan TJ, Styer PE, Mody DR. Bethesda 2001 implementation and reporting rates: 2003 practices of participants in the College of American Pathologists Interlaboratory Comparison Program in Cervicovaginal Cytology. *Arch Pathol Lab Med.* 2004;128(11):1224-1229.

11. Wright TC, Cox JT, Massad LS, Twiggs LB, Wilkinson EJ, for the 2001 ASCCP-Sponsored Consensus Conference. 2001 consensus guidelines for the management of women with cervical cytological abnormalities. *JAMA.* 2002;287:2120-2129.

12. Austin RM. Managing risk in gynecologic cytology: reactive and unsatisfactory smears. *Cancer.* 1997;81:137-138.

13. Davey DD, Woodhouse SL, Styer P, Stastny J, Mody D. Atypical epithelial cells and specimen adequacy: current laboratory practices of participants in the College of American Pathologists interlaboratory comparison program in cervicovaginal cytology. *Arch Pathol Lab Med.* 2000;124:203-211.

14. Tritz DM, Weeks JA, Spires SE, et al. Etiologies for non-correlating cervical cytologies and biopsies. *Am J Clin Pathol.* 1995;103:594-597.

15. Jones BA, Novis DA. Cervical biopsy-cytology correlation: a College of American Pathologist's Q-Probes study of 22439 correlations in 348 laboratories. *Arch Pathol Lab Med.* 1996;120:523-531.

16. Davey DD. Papanicolaou 5-year retrospective review: what is required by the Clinical Laboratory Improvement Amendments of 1988? *Arch Pathol Lab Med.* 1997;121:296-298.

17. Davey DD. Amended reports: when if ever? *Diagn Cytopathol.* 1997; 17:399-400.

18. Colgan TJ, Woodhouse SL, Styer P, Kennedy M, Davey DD. Reparative changes and the false-positive/false-negative Papanicolaou test: a study from the College of American Pathologists Interlaboratory Comparison Program in Cervicovaginal Cytology. *Arch Pathol Lab Med.* 2001;125:134-140.

19. Davey DD, Neilsen ML, Frable WJ, Rosenstock W, Lowell DM, Kraemer BB. Improving accuracy in gynecologic cytology: results of the College of American Pathologists Interlaboratory Comparison Program in Cervicovaginal Cytology (PAP). *Arch Pathol Lab Med.* 1993;117:1193-1198.

20. Woodhouse SL, Stastny J, Styer P, Kennedy M, Praestgaard AH, Davey DD. Interobserver variability in subclassification of squamous intraepithelial lesions: results of the College of American Pathologists Interlaboratory Comparison Program in Cervicovaginal Cytology. *Arch Pathol Lab Med.* 1999;123:1079-1084.

21. Jones BA. Rescreening in gynecologic cytology: rescreening of 8096 previous cases for current low-grade and indeterminate-grade squamous intraepithelial lesion diagnoses: a College of American Pathologists Q-Probes study of 323 laboratories. *Arch Pathol Lab Med.* 1996;120:519-522.

22. Jones BA, Novis DA. Follow-up of abnormal gynecologic cytology: a College of American Pathologists Q-Probes study of 16132 cases from 306 laboratories. *Arch Pathol Lab Med.* 2000;124:665-671.

23. Jones BA, Davey DD. Quality management in gynecologic cytology using interlaboratory comparison. *Arch Pathol Lab Med.* 2000;124:672-681.

24. Jones BA. Rescreening in gynecologic cytology. Rescreening of 3762 previous cases for current high-grade squamous intraepithelial lesion and carcinoma: a College of American Pathologists Q-Probes study of 312 institutions. *Arch Pathol Lab Med.* 1995;119:1097-1103.

25. Hatem F, Wilbur DC. High grade squamous cervical lesions following negative Papanicolaou smears: false-negative cervical cytology or rapid progression. *Diagn Cytopathol.* 1995;12:135-141.

26. Sherman ME, Kelly D. High-grade squamous intraepithelial lesions and invasive carcinoma following the report of three negative Papanicolaou smears: screening failures or rapid progression. *Mod Pathol.* 1992;5:377-342.

27. Austin RM. Follow-up of abnormal gynecologic cytology: a College of American Pathologists Q-Probes study of 16132 cases from 306 laboratories [editorial]. *Arch Pathol Lab Med.* 2000;124:1113-1114.

28. American Society of Cytopathology Statement on New Technologies in Cervical Cytology Screening. Available at: www.cytopathology.org/guidelines/guide_new_tech.php. Accessed March 3, 2005.

29. Intersociety Working Group for Cytology Technologies. Proposed guidelines for primary screening instruments for gynecologic cytology. *Acta Cytol.* 1997;41:924-934.

30. Austin RM, McLendon WW. The Papanicolaou smear: medicine's most successful cancer screening procedure is threatened. *JAMA.* 1997;277:754-755.

31. Fitzgibbons PL, Austin RM. Expert review of histologic slides and Papanicolaou tests in the context of litigation or potential litigation. *Arch Pathol Lab Med.* 2000;124:1717-1719.

32. American Society for Cytopathology. Guidelines for Review of Gyn Cytology Samples in the Context of Litigation or Potential Litigation. Available at: http://www.cytopathology.org/guidelines/index.php. Accessed March 3, 2005.

33. Abt AB, Abt LG, Olt GJ. The effect of interinstitution anatomic pathology consultation on patient care. *Arch Pathol Lab Med.* 1995;119:514-517.

34. Jones BA, Novis DA. Non-gynecologic cytology turnaround times: a College of American Pathologists Q-Probes study of 180 laboratories. *Arch Pathol Lab Med.* 2001;125:1279-1284.

35. Uniform approach to breast fine needle aspiration biopsy: a synopsis. *Acta Cytol.* 1996;40:1120-1126.

36. Woodman CL. What is informed? What is consent? What the cytopathologist needs to know. *Diagn Cytopathol.* 1998;19:1-3.

37. Chamberlain DW, Braude AC, Rebuck AS. A critical evaluation of bronchioalveolar lavage: criteria for identifying unsatisfactory specimens. *Acta Cytol.* 1987;31:599-605.

38. Guidelines of the Papanicolaou Society of Cytopathology for the examination of cytologic specimens obtained from the respiratory tract. *Mod Pathol.* 1999;12:427-436.

39. Guidelines of the Papanicolaou Society of Cytopathology for the examination of fine needle aspiration specimens from thyroid nodules. *Diagn Cytopathol.* 1996;15:84-89.

40. Kline TS. Adequacy and aspirates from the breast: a philosophical approach. *Diagn Cytopathol.* 1995;13:470-472.

41. Moriarty A. Fine-needle biopsy of the breast: when is enough, enough? *Diagn Cytopathol.* 1995;13:373-374.

42. Suen K, Kline TS, Nguyen G. Adequacy of non-gynecologic cell samples. In: *Critical Issues in Cytopathology.* New York: Igaku-Shoin; 1995:68-82.

43. Sidawy MK, Del Vecchio DM, Knoll SM. Fine needle aspiration biopsy of thyroid nodules: correlation between cytology and histology and evaluation of discrepant cases. *Cancer.* 1997;81:253-259.

Bibliography

Archives of Pathology & Laboratory Medicine. 1997;121:205-342. (March issue devoted to cytology quality and liability issues.)

CAP Guidelines for Review of Pap Tests in the Context of Litigation or Potential Litigation. Available at: http://www.cap.org:80/apps/docs/policies/policy_appZ.htm. Accessed March 3, 2005.

CAP PAP Interlaboratory Comparison Program in Cervicovaginal Cytopathology. Supplemental Questionnaire Results. Northfield, Ill: College of American Pathologists; 2004.

CAP PAP Interlaboratory Comparison Program in Cervicovaginal Cytopathology. 2003 PAP Year End Summary Report. Northfield, Ill: College of American Pathologists; 2003.

College of American Pathologists Strategic Science Symposium: human papillomavirus testing. *Arch Pathol Lab Med.* 2003;127:927-996.

College of American Pathologists. Laboratory Accreditation Program. Cytopathology Checklist. Available at: http://www.cap.org:80/apps/docs/laboratory_accreditation/checklists/checklistftp.html. Accessed March 3, 2005.

College of American Pathologists. Standards for Laboratory Accreditation. Available at: http://www.cap.org:80/apps/docs/laboratory_accreditation/standards/standards.html. Accessed March 3, 2005.

Council on Scientific Affairs. Quality assurance in cervical cytology: the Papanicolaou smear. *JAMA.* 1989;262:1672-1679.

Cytopathology Practice Committee, American Society of Cytopathology. Nongynecologic cytology practice guideline. *Acta Cytol.* 2004;48:521-546.

Improving the Quality of Clinician Pap Smear Technique and Management, Client Pap Smear Education, and the Evaluation of Pap Smear Laboratory Testing. Washington, DC: US Department of Health and Human Services, Public Health Service, Office of Family Planning; 1989.

Inhorn SL, Shalkham JE, Kurtycz DFI. Total quality management in cytology. *Acta Cytol.* 1993;37:261-266.

Kline TJ, Kline TS. Communication and cytopathology, part II: malpractice. *Diagn Cytopathol.* 1991;7:227-228.

Kline TS, Nguyen GK. *Critical Issues in Cytopathology.* New York: Igaku-Shoin; 1996.

Kline TS. The challenge of quality improvement with the Papanicolaou smear. *Arch Pathol Lab Med.* 1997;121:253-255.

Koss LG. Cervical (Pap) smear: new directions. *Cancer.* 1993;71:1406-1412.

Lachowicz C, Kline TS. Communication and cytopathology, part III: shared responsibility for quality improvement. *Diagn Cytopathol.* 1993;9:371-372.

Layfield LF, Elsheikh TM, Fili A, Nayar R, Shidham V. Review of the state of the art and recommendations of the Papanicolaou Society of Cytopathology for urinary cytology procedures and reporting: The Papanicolaou Society of Cytopathology Practice Guidelines Task Force. *Diagn Cytopathol.* 2004;30:24-30.

Merrick T, ed. *Laboratory Accreditation Manual.* Northfield, Ill: College of American Pathologists; 2003. Available at: http://www.cap.org:80/apps/cap.portal?_nfpb=true&_pageLabel=lab_accred_lab_info_page. Accessed March 3, 2005.

Mody DR, Davey DD, Branca M, et al. Quality assurance and risk reduction guidelines. *Acta Cytol.* 2000;44:496-507.

Nielsen ML. Cytopathology laboratory improvement programs of the College of American Pathologists Laboratory Accreditation Program (CAP LAP) and Performance Improvement Program in Cervicovaginal Cytology (CAP PAP). *Arch Pathol Lab Med.* 1997;121:256-259.

Solomon D, Davey D, Kurman R, et al. The 2001 Bethesda system: terminology for reporting the results of cervical cytology. *JAMA.* 2002;287:2114-2119.

Quality management in autopsy pathology

Mary Ann Sens, MD, PhD
Marcella Fierro, MD
Deborah Kay, MD

The autopsy consistently discovers unexpected findings and was recognized by the Institute of Medicine[1] as a rich, important, and underutilized quality assessment tool and opportunity for improvement of health care systems. A 1994 Q-Probes study by the College of American Pathologists[2] examined the performance of 2459 autopsies in 248 institutions, excluding all stillbirths and forensic cases. In this multi-institutional survey representing a broad cross-section of North American pathology practices, 40% of autopsies had at least one major clinically unexpected finding contributing to the patient's death, 17% had a minor finding contributing to death, and 32% a minor finding not contributing to death. A similar rate has been found in several other studies within selected institutions throughout the world,[3] in pediatric[4] and adult[5] populations. The frequency of unexpected findings has not changed significantly over time,[6,7] even with the advent of modern imaging and diagnostic techniques.

Autopsy studies have detailed many new disease entities. Legionnaires' disease, acquired immune deficiency syndrome (AIDS), Alzheimer's disease, hantavirus pulmonary syndrome (HPS), sudden infant death syndrome (SIDS), severe acute respiratory syndrome (SARS), and toxic shock syndrome are among the many diseases initially delineated through autopsies. The autopsy is the ultimate outcome data set[8] and a rich source of quality improvement information,[9] which can be readily incorporated into a quality management system.

A three-tiered systems approach to comprehensive quality management is critical to real and sustainable quality improvement. Checklists, which capture the essence of protocols and processes, create data for evidence-based quality evaluation systems. Benchmarking data analysis from the checklists creates opportunities for problem solving and improvements. Finally, continuous monitoring of the process identifies opportunities for systems enhancement, best practice incorporation, and insightful longitudinal analysis.

Autopsy quality assurance programs should cover all aspects of autopsy performance, from the preanalytic (permits, death investigation for forensic, communication, postmortem care), to analytic (performance of autopsy), and postanalytic (incorporation into hospital/system quality assurance program, clinical communication and review, court/medical-legal interface for forensic pathology) phases. The program must be individualized for the practice setting. Multi-year planning, with achievable and measurable annual goals, individualized to the institutional setting, is also needed as the program is implemented. External benchmarks should be used, when applicable, as well as incorporation of hospital/health system expectations and targeted improvement or assessment areas. Table 10-1 lists several model checklists and program activities to effectively and rapidly set up and monitor an autopsy quality assurance program in all areas of performance assessment. As programs are individualized, at least one metric from each area should be monitored in addition to standard turnaround times for autopsy components. Ideally, some metrics are maintained for several years to

Table 10-1. Performance assessment areas of autopsy quality assurance

Quality Control of Autopsy Processes
  Physical environment
  Permit completeness
  Postmortem care / death investigation
  Service performance expectations

Professional Assessment of Pathology / Autopsy / Laboratory Performance
  Gross demonstration and interpretation
  PAD to FAD correlation
  Photographic documentation
  Microscopic assessment
  Final assessment and interpretation
  Consult review
  Technical assessment of histology, ancillary testing

Clinical Communication and Correlation: Service Expectations from Consulting Physicians
  Correlation of clinical and autopsy diagnosis
  Correlation of cause of death from clinical and autopsy
  Communication through clinical conferences / other venues

Integrative Correlation of Autopsy Findings into Hospital / Health Care Improvements
  Cause-of-death vs non–cause-of-death
  Major and minor classification; VA, CAP or error classification
  Referral / correlation with tissue / M&M / peer-review institutional processes
  Integration into professional staffing re-credentialling processes
  Root cause analysis
  Referral to institutional committee / process, ie, infection control, professional staffing

Rates and Turnaround Times
  Autopsy rates for hospital / system; service / department; individual attending physician or team
  Technical turnaround times
  Autopsy turnaround times

obtain longitudinal data, while others are monitored for shorter periods and rechecked as desired. At least some of the autopsy metrics should reflect laboratory goals in quality management and be reported as such to quality committees of the institution. Table 10-2 lists temporal (preanalytic, analytic, postanalytic) and performance functions within the total quality management program.

Turnaround time

Turnaround times (TAT) for autopsy pathology must be maintained and reviewed as part of a quality management program. However, merely reporting turnaround time for the autopsy or select subcomponents (like the issuance of preliminary autopsy diagnosis [PAD]) does not reflect the total performance of an autopsy, nor can it identify sites of corrective action if targets are not met. Breakdown of the "steps" of an autopsy as they occur between laboratory divisions (clerical, technical, and professional) is extremely useful, especially when coupled to information readily

Table 10-2. Autopsy quality management scheme

	QC Processes	QA Pathology	QA Clinical Communication	QI Integration
Preanalytic	Autopsy permit Postmortem care Physical plant		Chart review, clinical communication Family/other communication	Service expectations: Funeral homes Clinicians Others (police, study protocols)
Analytic	Turnaround times	Gross findings Microscopic Ancillary testing	Clinical presence at autopsy	Case directed best practice protocol
Postanalytic	Postautopsy care	Correlation to previous pathology Correlation to other testing	CPC, M&M Informal communication Family/other communication	Organ or diagnosis review Physician/service review Clinical diagnosis review

obtained through laboratory information systems. Internal compilation of the turnaround time of individual processes within the autopsy will assist in identifying targets for improvement. For example, are prolonged histology turnaround times causing overall autopsy delays? Are pathologists with long dictation delays having more quality assurance problems with omitted diagnoses? What is the actual turnaround time for consultations such as neuropathology? Without the metrics of each step, identifying areas for improvement is more difficult. Breaking the overall turnaround time into individual steps, reviewing for improvement at each segment, and engaging the people involved in each process assists in the team-building concept and leads to autopsy improvement.

An example of a possible checklist for the individual turnaround time for components of the autopsy process is given in Table 10-3. Individual laboratories may have a laboratory information system to extract this data automatically, and individual units such as histology may desire to maintain a running turnaround time for all cases submitted. All can be utilized to track components of the total turnaround time for autopsy pathology.

Sample checklists and components: technical and quality control of autopsy

A number of checklists are included at the end of this chapter to aid in the assessment of technical and quality control of the autopsy process. An individual program may select one or more of these checklists, modify as needed for their organization, and track data for a defined period. If problems are consistently noted in a portion of the organization or process, these checklists may serve as valuable tools for root cause analysis. When an acceptable and stable performance is achieved, other checklists may be substituted in the quality assurance program, and the original checklist only sporadically monitored for continued performance.

Autopsy permit (Checklist 10-1). A guideline for the assessment of accuracy and completeness of autopsy permits. This may be used to assess the integrity of the consent process.

Postmortem care (Checklists 10-2a and 10-2b). These two checklists may be used to assess appropriate postmortem care of patients: one applicable to all deceased patients regardless of whether an autopsy is performed, the second for patients following the performance of an autopsy.

Autopsy/morgue facility (Checklist 10-3). This may be modified for individual facility needs, ie, include all supplies routinely utilized in the particular autopsy practice so that room and facility are well kept and maintained. Many of these items in the checklist reflect accreditation standards of the College of American Pathologists Laboratory Accreditation Program.

Histology technical review (Checklist 10-4). This may be used to assess histology processes for autopsy cases and may be incorporated into histology laboratory quality control.

Photography imaging review (Checklist 10-5). This may be used to assess the technical quality of photographs or digital images taken at autopsy as well as the accurate representation of gross findings.

Sample checklists and components: professional quality assurance in autopsy

These checklists assess the performance, review, and interpretations of the autopsy. They may be incorporated into departmental quality assurance programs of pathology practice. This assessment is common in other areas of anatomic pathology but is scantly discussed for autopsy pathology.[10] It is vitally important, particularly if clinical correlation and assessment is done, that professional assessment and standards within pathology practice are met.

Gross dissection and examination (Checklist 10-6). Due to wide variety of practices (large university training programs to solo/small group community hospital practices), modification of the checklist to suit practice patterns is needed. However, some assessment of the gross interpretations should be included in an autopsy quality assurance program in all settings.

Organ-specific evaluation (Checklist 10-7). There is also value in a detailed checklist for specific organ examination, which may be used selectively. This is an example for evaluating the gross and microscopic examination of the heart. Laboratories may wish to develop other checklists for other organ systems as part of the Quality Performance Assessment.

Microscopic assessment (Checklist 10-8). Evaluation of microscopic assessment in autopsy pathology parallels programs in surgical pathology and cytology. This checklist may be used for programs focused on autopsy pathology, or microscopic assessment may be included within other departmental quality assurance activities focused on microscopic interpretations and diagnosis

Ancillary testing/suitability (Checklist 10-9). This may be used to evaluate the frequency and utility of ancillary tests in autopsy pathology.

Consultative services (no checklist). All intradepartmental and external consultations should be documented for autopsy pathology within the report and within an existing consultative quality assurance program. This mirrors the consultative practice in surgical pathology and cytology. A separate checklist is not included, but laboratories should include autopsy consultation in the departmental quality assurance programs.

Preliminary autopsy diagnosis and final autopsy diagnosis comparison (Checklist 10-10). This is a useful comparison, particularly in the training of residents and pathologists' assistants. Complete concordance is not expected; however, the exercise provides the opportunities for participants to sharpen gross diagnostic skills.

Table 10-3. Turnaround times: case-based format

Case ID: Date: Pathologist: Resident: Student:	Date Done	Date Returned (if applicable)	Times	Variance or Comment
Gross dissection		N/A		
Histology submission			TAT histology:	
Special stains			TAT specials:	
Supplemental submission			TAT supplemental:	
PAD written				
PAD transcribed				
PAD to clinicians			TAT PAD: (from date of autopsy)	
Other PAD metric				
Histology review				
Histology review with attending				
Gross dictation done			TAT gross: (from date of autopsy)	
Gross dictation transcribed				
Neuropathology consultation				
Brain cutting				
Neuro histology				
Neuropathology report			TAT neuro:	
Final correlation				
Final dictation done				
Final dictation transcribed				
Final corrections				
Final completed				
Final to clinicians / others			Autopsy TAT: (from date of autopsy)	

Random total case review (Checklist 10-11). A random total case review may provide additional and integrative information regarding the performance of an autopsy. This checklist provides for the review of all case aspects of an autopsy.

Sample checklists and components: communication

Communication before, during, and after an autopsy is vital among concerned parties to assure that the goals of an autopsy are achieved, and should be included in an autopsy quality assurance program. Several checklists are provided to document and improve this aspect of autopsy practice. Depending on the practice, additional individuals or organizations may also be included in this activity. For example, forensic practices may include police and investigators; trauma centers may include field personnel and referring hospitals. All checklists should be modified to suit individual practice needs.

Preautopsy review of clinical information and autopsy participation (Checklist 10-12). This evaluates the effectiveness and completeness of communication prior to and during the performance of an autopsy.

Postautopsy clinical communication (Checklist 10-13). This checklist documents the variety of mechanisms of communication of autopsy results.

Family and other communication (Checklist 10-14). This checklist documents communication with parties other than the clinical care team. These may include families, courts, police, referring hospitals, emergency medical field personnel, or organ procurement organizations.

Sample checklists and components: quality integration of autopsy

Case-specific clinical and autopsy diagnosis comparison and correlation

Every autopsy should have correlation of clinical and autopsy findings. Several models to conduct this comparison have been described. The exact method used may be facilitated or handicapped by flexibility of information and reporting systems used in autopsy performance. A summary of the classifications used and a recommendation for alternative systems is given.

CAP classification

The CAP proposed a classification of autopsy and clinical diagnosis in a simple form, filled out for each case (Table 10-4). This classification is used in some pathology practices for individual case evaluation (Table 10-5). The shortcomings of this evaluation tool include the lack of definitions of the categories, leaving a somewhat subjective interpretation of categories. Clinical input to the process varies dramatically between institutions, occasionally creating difficulty in validation of reporting.

VA classification

A different model for error classification at autopsy is in use in VA hospitals. It is similar to the CAP classification in that judgments are made with regard to "major" and "minor" findings and whether conditions were significant or alternate treatment opportunities existed if diagnoses were known prior to death. The advantage of this system is its use throughout the VA hospital system and its uniformity of classification with clinical care reviews within the VA system.

Cause-of-death related classification

This system focuses on classification of diagnoses that contribute to death, rather than delineating all autopsy and clinical diagnoses. Diagnoses are classified as to whether they contributed to the patient's death or not. Generally this is less subjective and more likely to reach concordance in clinical correlations. This scheme also gives valuable insight into problems associated with cause-of-death determination without an autopsy. Although truly minor medical conditions are aggregated into more significant underlying medical conditions that may not have caused death, this classification scheme does avoid some subjective assessments with "major" and "minor" groupings. This also avoids the subjective and occasionally contentious judgments as to potential treatment options or possible clinical course alteration.

ICD coding

Discharge diagnoses are nearly uniformly coded by health systems, resulting in a numeric-based reporting of diagnostic information. Autopsy diagnosis can be similarly coded, creating an opportunity for more automated comparison of autopsy and clinical diagnosis. This holds promise for autopsy studies. It also avoids classification of the diagnostic differences between autopsy and clinical studies into "major," "minor," and treatment options. Additionally, this type of scheme, focusing on disease entity review, tends to be system-oriented and may be used for targeted error analysis and action. This scheme may be combined with cause-of-death related classification for further data analysis.

Autopsy report formatting to facilitate clinical correlation

Simple formatting of autopsy reports into a two-column listing of clinical diagnosis with corresponding (or not) autopsy diagnosis facilitates review and classification of autopsy findings. A simple format for comparison of clinical and autopsy diagnosis, with or without the assistance of ICD coding, is given in Checklist 10-15.

Case-specific review and incorporation into institutional quality assurance programs

Correlation of autopsy and clinical diagnosis should be reported or reviewed by institutional quality assurance committees. The exact mechanisms may vary depending on the organization; however, this information may be reported to entities, such as a tissue committee, peer-review committee, morbidity and mortality committee, QA coordinator, or various practice teams that are charged with oversight of clinical practice. While the mechanism and reporting format will be dependent on organizational structure, pathology quality assurance programs have the responsibility for distribution of this type of information to appropriate committees beyond the laboratory.

Cumulative review of cases

The composite review of cases is a valuable contribution of autopsy quality assurance and some procedure should be devised to accomplish it. Table 10-4 gives a cumulative reporting format for a community hospital with a low number of autopsies, using the individual case assessment derived from the CAP data set. In this study, 3 years of autopsy CAP forms were tabulated for the Medical Executive QA Report, shown in the table as years 1 through 3. All deaths at this hospital had been reviewed, with the completed CAP form for each autopsy (Table 10-5), as part of the hospital quality assurance activities, and in each case of potential discrepancy, the standard of care for that case was thought to been met. However, the cumulative 3-year review revealed that four of the "unsuspected" diagnoses were cardiac in nature, and although benchmarking data was not available

Table 10-4. Community Hospital "X": autopsy summary review form

Calendar Year	Year 1	% Cases	Year 2	% Cases	Year 3	% Cases	Year 4	% Cases
# Autopsies performed	19		15		13		13	
# Autopsies with clinical records	15		10		9		11	
# Autopsies that uncovered a major disagreement in diagnosis	3	20	3	30	2	22	5	45
# Discrepant diagnosis with possible adverse impact on survival	0		2	20	1	11	1	9
# Discrepant diagnosis with equivocal impact on survival	4	15	3	30	1	11	4	36
# Discrepant secondary disease (symptomatic)			0					
# Discrepant occult secondary disease	1	5	1	10	3	33	3	27
# Autopsies that establish unexpected or additional diagnosis	8	53	7	70	6	67	6	55
# Autopsies with potential different clinical outcome, if known	0		2	20			0	
# Autopsies providing clarification of differential diagnosis	10	67	6	60	6	67	7	64
# Autopsies confirming or verifying major diagnosis	9	60	7	70	7	78	7	64
# Autopsies providing information on treatment effects	3	20	2	20	4	44	6	55
# Autopsies providing information on diagnostic procedures (radiologic, endoscopic, other)	0		0		3	33	5	45
# Autopsies providing information on pathology diagnostic procedures	1	7	0		5	56	3	27
# Autopsies with additional coding possible*	6	40	5	50	4	44	**	**

* Not on original CAP checklist; added for hospital study

** Medical records incorporate autopsy findings

Approved by: _____

Date: _____

Committee Comments: *(Deleted for confidentiality in peer review)*

Table 10-5: Case analysis for year 4

Cases with Possible Impact of Care (CAP Classification):

Case: AYY-XXX   Discrepant diagnosis: Acute myocardial infarction

Clinical – Autopsy Discrepancy: Not recognized clinically

Pathology review discrepancy: Autopsy pathologist estimated time course at 1–2 days; review of slides demonstrate MI 5–10 days old with possible acute (hours) extension.

Clinical Setting: Admission 7 days prior to death in 85-year-old female. Admit dx UTI, CHF, possible pneumonia. Elevated WBC; febrile, abnormal EKG, elevated CKMB, abnormal U/A; bacteria/WBC, culture positive. Treated with Ab for UTI. Expired suddenly prior to transfer back to nursing home.

Assessment by Pathology QA:
1. Equivocal impact for particular patient, who was DNR and moribund; family likely would have refused additional treatment if diagnosis made. However, a possible adverse impact for apparent non-recognition of AMI by admitting physician; referred to peer review committee.
2. Peer review of myocardial infarction dating with autopsy pathologist.

One action of the hospital review committee was to do a root cause analysis of this incident. System findings included:
1. Poor information flow with testing ordered in ER, resulted when patient on floor.
2. Poor information flow between ER physicians, shift change and admitting physician
3. Potential contribution from "automatic" reading of EKG instrumentation.

These issues were addressed by appropriate individuals and teams with modification of procedures to enhance patient care. In addition, counseling for the pathologist originally estimating dates of the AMI was accomplished.

AYY-XXX: Pulmonary embolus in 36 year old woman. Age, lack of risk factors and suddenness of onset raised possible genetic coagulopathy. Family physician notified for possible evaluation of other family members.

No impact on immediate patient care outcome *saddle embolus, catastrophic; review of available medical history without clear indication of previous coagulopathy; possible major care implication for family members.

Follow-up: Genetic related coagulopathy in some family members; major care implications for family members.

Equivocal Impact:

AYY-XXX: Patient with history of lung Ca; admitted for abdominal pain; rapid deterioration. Unsuspected residual Ca and acute bronchopneumonia at autopsy; autopsy limited to chest only.

Minimal /Equivocal impact. Cause of abdominal symptoms still not clear due to autopsy restrictions.

AYY-XXX: Progressive dementia, etiology not clear; neuropathology at autopsy demonstrated a progressive supranuclear palsy.

No impact on patient outcome.

Family reassured with elimination of other causes of premature dementia.

AYY-XXX: Patient with hx of prostatic ca and 1.5 cm renal mass, benign on PET scan. Patient was at increased risk for renal surgery; elected to observe lesion. Eight months later, a poorly differentiated carcinoma, metastatic lesions found, uncertain origin. Patient expired within two months, RCC present at autopsy, no other site for primary determined. Renal mass unchanged in interval within imaging error.

Equivocal impact on patient outcome; assessment of previous diagnostic testing.

Changes in physician usage of PET data and interpretation.

for this occurrence, the incidence seemed high and had not been suspected with the individual case review. This finding lent support to the request for more monitored beds in the institution. An additional finding of this initial 3-year study demonstrated that re-coding of the discharge diagnosis to more accurately reflect diagnoses at autopsy revealed improvement in coding accuracy. This resulted in a policy change within the hospital to incorporate these findings routinely in all autopsied patients. Continuation of this computation in year 4 was accompanied by case analysis and comments (with deletion of peer review findings). Again, analysis of the autopsy findings proved a valuable contribution to the quality assurance programs, even at this small hospital with relatively low autopsy rates. It should also be noted that the most useful information resulted when discrepancies were cumulatively reviewed and classified by type, eg, are myocardial infarctions being missed, followed by a root cause analysis of variations.

Organ-based or diagnostic-based review, multiple cases

Trending or review of diagnostically related entities,[11] such as all pulmonary emboli, undiagnosed cancer, myocardial infarctions, etc, may be a useful review of autopsy studies.[9] It is suggested that a single disease grouping or patient population be examined in a QA cycle and, if indicated, patient care system improvement be addressed. This is also useful in the forensic setting, where diagnostic and investigational criteria should be established for an "ideal" investigation of a particular forensic entity, such as for SIDS or gunshot wounds; then reviewed cases are compared against the established metrics. With some planning, these organ-based or patient-population-based reviews may coincide with complimentary system reviews of processes. For example, detailed review of heart findings (for assessment of pathology), cardiac related deaths (for the system), and coronary artery bypass graft (CABG) patients could coincide with input as the system reviews cardiac diagnosis related groups (DRGs) or cardiothoracic surgeon performance.

Service-based review, multiple cases

Evaluation by clinical service, such as neonatal, CABG patients, pneumonia, etc, can contribute to existing hospital and system-based review. Most organizations have defined review cycles for physicians, DRGs, or procedures. Planning the autopsy review to contribute to these existing examinations harnesses the synergy and resources of the institution in the departmental quality assurance programs.

Additional activities for quality improvement

In addition to laboratory-based analysis, surveys of potential clients (eg, clinicians, funeral homes, organ procurement agencies) regarding the autopsy service may be of assistance. Since there is such a broad range of practices and issues, specific checklists or examples are not given, since they need to be individualized to an institution and clients. However, a short, three- to four-question, "How are we doing? Can we be doing things better? What is important to you?," to physicians, ER and ward personnel, and funeral homes will provide great insight to local issues. More importantly, it sends the strong message of commitment to excellence in service that is the goal of quality assurance programs. An annual or bi-annual survey of a targeted group is one sign of a well functioning quality assurance program.

Table 10-6. Data sets for autopsy correlation and quality improvement activities

Identifiable Information
    ID:
    Name:
    SS#:
    MRN#:
    Other identifiable information, if desired:
    Linking number (generated and linked to the data set stripped of ID):

Stripped Data Set
    Linking ID:
    Birth date:
    Age:
    Age units:
    Sex:
    Race:
    Ethnicity:
    Physician data (may be coded if physician codes are used in institution):
        Primary or referring physician:
        Admitting physician:
        Surgeon:
        Other physicians:
    Service(s):
    Procedures:
    Surgery(ies):
    LOS (length of stay):

Data Set for Correlation
    Admission ICD codes:
    Clinical major discharge code (or cause of death):
    Additional clinical discharge code:
    Autopsy cause of death code:
    Additional autopsy diagnostic codes:

Information systems, database development, and de-identified data sets

Additional metrics are valuable in autopsy quality assurance programs and allow for quality improvement opportunities and longitudinal assessment of cases. These are highly suited for data sets with the significant bulk of information in a patient de-identified data set. This allows more objective comparisons and concentrates efforts at system issues, rather than individual case idiosyncrasies. It also creates a more positive and less confrontational approach to potential errors and encourages a systems-based quality improvement program.

Table 10-6 gives some examples of data sets and de-identified information that may be more broadly used in autopsy analysis. If hospital and laboratory information systems or customized database development are used for quality assurance programs, incorporation of these metrics will give flexibility to the system in final analysis.

On many autopsy suites, the Latin phrase, "This is the place that death delights to serve the living," is displayed. Autopsy studies, both hospital-based and forensic, can provide the quality standard for health care delivery, emerging injury and disease patterns, and an objective basis for medical-legal investigation and jurisprudence. The implementation of quality assessment and improvement practices in autopsy practice will enable this service to the living.

Index of checklists

Checklist 10-1. Autopsy permit

Objective: To document accuracy and completeness of autopsy permits and identify opportunities for improvement in consenting for autopsy.

Dates of data collection:

Form return to:

Case / ID: Date:	Satisfactory	Problem Noted	Comment
Was permit signed by next of kin (NOK)?			
Was permit signed by MD or other authorized requester?			
Was permit witnessed?			
Were limitations noted?			
Was a contact necessary to clarify any part of permit?			
Was clinical information desired by physician requesting autopsy noted on permit (when available on form)?			
Were family specific questions or information noted on permit form?			
Was clinical contact information present on form?			
Was identified NOK correct?			
Was pathology notified in acceptable time frame?			
Permit by telephone _____ in person _____			
Did permit issues require contact or resigning of permit? If yes, explain in Comment.			

Data analysis:

Checklist 10-2a. Postmortem care (prior to autopsy/no autopsy done)

Objective: To document postmortem care of patient.

Dates of data collection:

Form return to:

Case / ID: Date:	Yes – Satisfactory	No – Problem Noted	Comment
Was body shrouded completely?			
Did positioning minimize lividity to hands, face?			
Were tubes removed?			
Should tubes have been left in place?			
Was soft material used to position hands?			
Was body identified with wrist band?			
Was body identified with toe tag?			
Was exterior of shroud marked or tagged with body?			
Was body logged into morgue?			
Other postmortem care problems?			
Was adhesive tape removed from visible portions of body?			
Lip protection, moisture used?			
Eyes closed?			
Were personal effects on body inventoried?			
Were personal effects not on body inventoried and with body or in secure location?			

Checklist 10-2b. Postmortem care (after autopsy)

Objective: To document postmortem care of patient following autopsy.

Dates of data collection:

Form return to:

Case / ID: Date:	Yes – Satisfactory	No – Problem Noted	Comment
Was body cleaned?			
Was body shrouded completely?			
Did positioning minimize lividity to hands, face?			
Was soft material used to position hands?			
Was body identified with toe tag?			
Was exterior of shroud marked or tagged with body?			
Was body logged into morgue?			
Other postmortem care problems?			
Was adhesive tape removed from visible portions of body?			
Lip protection, moisture used?			
Eyes closed?			
Were personal effects on body inventoried?			
Were personal effects not on body inventoried and with body or in secure location?			
Was funeral home notified in acceptable time frame?			
Was body logged out of morgue?			

Checklist 10-3. Autopsy/morgue facility

Objective: To provide regular evaluation of physical environment of morgue/autopsy suite to meet laboratory set standards of performance.

Dates of data collection:

Form return to:

Date:
Person completing form:

	Satisfactory	Not Satisfactory	Comments; Corrective Action	CAP Checklist (if applicable)
Items				
Linens				
Gowns, protective equipment				
Instruments				
Disposable blades				
Blood/fluid tubes and containers				
Storage containers				
Microbiologic materials				
Formalin				
Body charts and diagrams				
Pens, pencils				
Cassettes				
Procedure manuals				ANP.02888
DNA cards				
Environmental				
Room cleanliness				
Instruments – cleanliness				
Morgue temperature				
Lighting				ANP.11300
Odors noted				ANP.11300 ANP.11350
Formalin monitor data				ANP.08216
Dictation space/supplies				ANP.11400
Photography space/supplies				ANP.11450

Checklist 10-4. Histology, technical

Objective: To evaluate slide preparation for an autopsy case. Separate assessments by the technologist, technologist QA person and the pathologists. Information is also obtained regarding grossing skills of person submitting slides to the laboratory and serves as a portion of gross examination QA.

Dates of data collection:

Form return to:

Case / ID: Date:	Satisfactory	Problem Noted	Comment
Assessment by Technologist			
Were cassettes labeled sequentially and correctly?			(refer to grossing QA)
Were sections of satisfactory thickness and size?			(refer to grossing QA)
Were sections fixed properly?			(refer to grossing QA)
Assessment of Technical Product by QA Technologist			
Are sections embedded correctly?			
Are knife marks or tears present?			
Is staining satisfactory?			
Dehydration problems?			
Is coverslipping satisfactory?			
Technical problems noted?			
Assessment of Technical Product by Pathologist			
Is embedding satisfactory?			
Is staining satisfactory?			
Are slides of diagnostic quality?			

Checklist 10-5. Photography, imaging

Objective: To provide assessment of the use of photography in the autopsy.

> Note: Institutions should decide if and how much photography should be used in the autopsy. This may range from complete documentation of external and gross internal findings (positive and negative), to selected and optional photographs. This checklist assumes optional and selective use of photographs to document significant gross findings of sufficient quality to present at a case review or clinical conference. If complete photographic documentation is desired, this checklist should be expanded. If participants prefer a more technically oriented checklist, more photographic information may be included. There is wide regional and institutional variation regarding identity issues and use of autopsy photographs. Programs must be familiar with state laws and institutional policy regarding autopsy photography.

Dates of data collection:

Form return to:

Case / ID: Date:	Yes	No	Reason
Were gross findings documented by photography/images?			
Was lighting balanced and sufficient to demonstrate findings?			
Were there distractions in the photograph (extraneous blood, utensils, debris, glare from flash or lighting)?			
Was the desired finding in focus?			
Did the image demonstrate the desired finding?			
Was a scale needed and used?			
Do colors within photograph appear natural and balanced?			
Do identification issues in photos conform to institutional policy and state law?			

Checklist 10-6. Gross dissection and examination

Objective: To assess gross examination completeness, compliance with autopsy permit and gross diagnosis accuracy, to identify opportunities for improvement in gross diagnostic ability.

Dates of data collection:

Form return to:

	Review of Organs and Body Prior to Release	Review of Organs/Photos But Not Body	Review of Report and Sections
Type of Review:			
Case / ID: **Date:**	Yes	Problem Noted	Comment
Where autopsy limitations adhered to?			
Did dissection demonstrate findings adequately?			
Was optimal approach used to demonstrate findings?			
Was exterior of body adequately described?			
Were organ relationships and body cavity adequately described?			
Were weights taken, as appropriate?			
Were measurements taken, as appropriate?			
Were organs described in enough detail to support positive findings?			
Were organs described in enough detail to support negative findings?			
Did gross organ findings correlate with diagnosis in PAD?			
Did microscopic findings support gross descriptions and diagnosis?			
Were problems noted with submission of gross tissue (Histology checklist)?			
Were sections submitted to adequately support gross diagnosis?			

Checklist 10-7. Organ-specific evaluations: examples for gross and microscopic heart examination

Objective: To provide detailed assessment of heart examination at autopsy.

Note: This may be most useful in a teaching setting or as a focused review in a non-teaching setting when correlated and used as an information base with a system wide review of cardiovascular deaths, CV services, or CV practitioners.

Dates of data collection:

Form return to:

Case / ID: Date: Pathologist:	Satisfactory	Other	Comment
Was the heart weighed?			
Comment on configuration (normal, globoid)			
Comment on ventricular size/dilatation? Thickness?			
Description of pericardial sac?			
Comment on fluid in pericardial sac?			
Major vessel attachment?			
Description epicardial surface?			
Method of dissection appropriate for expected findings?			
Would another method of dissection revealed more findings or more readily demonstrated pathology?			
Course, description of coronary arteries?			
Estimation of coronary artery disease and location?			
Description of coronary ostia?			
Description of myocardium?			
Location of any myocardial lesions?			
Description of endocardium?			
Examination for VSD, ASD?			
Comment on mural thrombi?			
Measurement of valves?			
Description of valves?			
Description of papillary muscle?			
Other pertinent gross finding?			
Special dissection needed?			
Special dissection done?			

Case / ID: Date: Pathologist:	Satisfactory	Other	Comment
Number of sections appropriate for gross findings?			
Microscopic findings correlation with gross?			
Assessment of microscopic findings?			
Special stains desired?			
Speclial stains done?			
Final diagnosis correlated in report?			
Final diagnosis correlation to clinical diagnosis?			

Listing of CV Diagnosis

Clinical	Autopsy	Agreement	Comment

Checklist 10-8. Microscopic assessment

Objective: To evaluate microscopic assessment within autopsy pathology. This may be done blindly
              or as part of a case review.

Directions: Blind review: All microscopic slides are given to a reviewing pathologist. The reviewing
              pathologist lists microscopic diagnosis and these are compared to autopsy microscopic findings.

              Case review: All case materials are provided to the reviewing pathologist

Dates of data collection:

Form return to:

Case / ID:

Date:

Slide	Reviewing Pathology Diagnosis	Agreement

For Case Directed Review:

Autopsy Diagnosis	Reviewing Pathology Diagnosis	Agreement; Comments

Checklist 10-9. Ancillary testing and suitability review

Objective: Ancillary testing (chemistry, microbiology, x-rays, special dissections, such as air embolism demonstration, osmium fixation of tissue slides, AV node dissection, or other deviation from standard technique) can enhance case findings when judiciously used. This checklist consists of two forms, one for the review of ancillary testing in a given case; the other a cumulative tally of specific ancillary testing method.

Dates of data collection:

Form return to:

Case / ID: Date	Yes	Problem Noted	Comment
Were chemistry/laboratory testing done postmortem?			
What testing was done?			
Would chemistry testing been helpful in case assessment?			
Were blood/urine other fluid held for possible testing?			
Would holding fluids have been helpful?			
Were radiographs done?			
If yes, did they contribute to case?			
If no, would they have assisted in case?			
Radiographs taken:			
Were microbiologic testing done?			
What type microbiologic testing done?			
If yes, did they contribute to case?			
If no, would they have assisted in case?			
Were special dissections done?			
If yes, did they contribute to case?			
What special dissection / demonstration was done			
If no, would they have assisted in case?			
What special dissection may have assisted?			

Ancillary technique log for each laboratory section:

Laboratory testing area _____ (microbiology, chemistry, toxicology, x-ray)

Test*	Case	Result	Assisted in Case**

 * Ancillary testing; each laboratory section should keep their own log; the exact test (ie, aerobic blood culture, swab cultures, viral culture etc) should be listed along with case, result and assessment, from the Ancillary QA form, as to the usefulness of the test.

** As determined from the preceding ancillary QA form.

Checklist 10-10. PAD and FAD correlation

Objective: To assess the correlation between PAD and FAD in autopsy practice. This is a measure of gross diagnostic accuracy.

The PAD are listed and, at the time of microscopic review and formulation of the FAD, the reviewing pathologist assesses if there was agreement between the PAD and FAD, and if not, if such was expected for the disease process.

Dates of data collection:

Form return to:

Case / ID:

Date:

Prosector: **Student** _____ **Resident** _____ **year** _____

Reviewing Pathologist:

Preliminary Autopsy Diagnosis (PAD)	Final Autopsy Diagnosis (FAD)	Agreement	Expectations / Comment

Checklist 10-11. Total pathology case review

Objective: This form serves as a concise case review, covering gross, microscopic and integrative findings of an autopsy. It may be particularly useful as an ongoing "random" case review in a departmental QA process.

Dates of data collection:

Form return to:

Case / ID: Date:	Yes	No – Problem Encountered	Comment (applicable CAP checklist item noted)
Were autopsy limitations adhered to?			
Are final diagnosis supported by gross and microscopic findings?			
Are photos or images of case demonstrative of findings?			
Do gross descriptions and dissections appear complete?			
Is microscopic assessment of case complete and accurate?			
Are there additional diagnoses on review?			
Are special stains and ancillary testing appropriate?			
Was report readable, clear and useful?			
Was consultation obtained and documented?			ANP.30050
Was external consultation obtained and documented?			ANP.10200
Other comments:			

Checklist 10-12. Preautopsy review of clinical information

Objective: To evaluate the effectiveness and utility clinical communication prior to an autopsy.

Dates of data collection:

Form return to:

Case / ID: Date:	Yes	No	Comment
Was MD requester contacted prior to autopsy?			
Was chart available prior to autopsy?			
Was chart reviewed prior to autopsy?			
Were other clinicians contacted prior to autopsy?			Who, when, why:
Did clinician or team attend portion of autopsy?			Team members present:
Was additional clinical information obtained by contact?			
Were goals or autopsy limitations clarified by contact?			
Other comments regarding preautopsy clinical communication			

Checklist 10-13. Postautopsy review of clinical information

Objective: To evaluate the extent and effectiveness of clinical exchange of information learned from autopsies and to improve correlation of autopsy and clinical diagnosis.

Dates of data collection:

Form return to:

Case / ID: Date:	Yes	No	Comments
Was clinician called at conclusion of the autopsy?			
Was the PAD sent?			
Was a consultation letter to the clinician sent at conclusion of autopsy?			
Was there a mutual review of clinical correlation with autopsy findings?			
Did clinical team input to correlation with autopsy findings?			
Was presentation of findings done in clinical conference? (M&M, CPC, sectional or departmental conference)			List conferences:

Checklist 10-14. Family and other communication

Objective: To evaluate the extent and effectiveness of communication to individuals other than clinicians requesting the autopsy. This form may be modified for other types of communication, eg, police and court for forensic cases, external hospitals referring cases, field EMS units, or other entities requiring information from an autopsy.

Dates of data collection:

Form return to:

Case / ID:

Date:

	Yes	No	Comment
Did family request communication regarding autopsy results?			
Did family obtain results?	Method: Call ____ Letter ____ Electronic ____ Face-to-face ____ Through clinician ____ Conference with clinician ____ Other _____		Date of communication: What was result of communication?

Checklist 10-15. Clinical diagnosis and autopsy diagnosis correlation table

Code*	Clinical Cause of Death	Autopsy Cause of Death	Code*	Agree**
Discharge Diagnostic Codes*	**Clinical Problem List**	**Pathology Correlation**	**Autopsy Diagnostic Codes***	**Agree***
Code*	**Clinical Cause of Death**	**Autopsy Cause of Death**	**Code***	**Agree***
Discharge Diagnostic Codes*	**Clinical Problem List**	**Pathology Correlation**	**Autopsy Diagnostic Codes***	**Agree***

* Autopsy and clinical diagnostic codes may be ICD, SNOMED, or other numeric classification disease code entities. The use of standard coding, such as ICD, allows abstractors and coders to perform this function, allowing ready comparison of clinical and autopsy diagnosis.

**Agreement codes:
TP: True positive – disease suspected clinically and confirmed with autopsy
FP: False positive – disease suspected clinically but not present at autopsy
TN: True negative – disease eliminated from clinical consideration and not present at autopsy
FN: False negative – disease not thought clinically but present at autopsy
N/C: No correlation expected; clinical entity without anatomic correlate (eg, hypotension, depression)
N/A: Site not examined at autopsy (usually related to permit restrictions)

References

1. Washington AE, McDonald KM, Kaveh G, Shojania KG, Burton EC, Goldman L. The autopsy as an outcome and performance measure. *Evid Rep Technol Assess (Summ)*. 2002;58:1-5.

2. Zarbo RJ, Baker PB, Howanitz PJ. The autopsy as a performance measurement tool-diagnostic discrepancies and unresolved clinical questions: a College of American Pathologists Q-Probes study of 2479 autopsies from 248 institutions. *Arch Pathol Lab Med*. 1999;123:191-198.

3. Grundmann E. Autopsy as a clinical quality control: A study of 15,143 cases. *In Vivo*. 1994;8:945-949.

4. Cartidge PH, Dawson AT, Stewart JH, Vujanic GM. Value and quality of perinatal and infant postmortem examinations: cohort analysis of 400 consecutive deaths. *BMJ*. 1995;21:155-158.

5. Stevanovic G, Tucakovic G, Dotlic R, Kanjuh V. Correlation of clinical diagnosis with autopsy findings: a retrospective study of 2,145 consecutive autopsies. *Hum Pathol*. 1986;17:1225-1230.

6. Kirch W, Schafil C. Misdiagnosis at a university hospital in 4 medical eras. *Medicine*. 1996;75:29-40.

7. Shojania KG, Burton EC, McDonald KM, Goldman L. Changes in rates of autopsy-detected diagnostic errors over time: a systematic review. *JAMA*. 2003;289:2849-2956.

8. Anderson RE, Hill RB, Gorstein F. A model for autopsy based quality assessment of medical diagnostics. *Hum Pathol*. 1990;21:174-181.

9. Hill RB, Anderson RE. An autopsy-based quality assessment program for improvement of diagnostic accuracy. *Qual Assur Health Care*. 1993;5:351-359.

10. Veress B, Gadaleanu V, Nennessmo I, Wilstrom BM. The reliability of autopsy diagnostics: inter-observer variation between pathologists, a preliminary report. *Qual Assur Health Care*. 1993;5:333-337.

11. Saracci, R. Problems with the use of autopsy results as a yardstick in the medical audit and epidemiology. *Qual Assur Health Care*. 1993;5:339-344.

Glossary

ACS-CoC	American College of Surgeons Commission on Cancer
ADASP	Association of Directors of Anatomic and Surgical Pathology
AGC	Atypical glandular cells
AIDS	Acquired immunodeficiency syndrome
AP	Anatomic pathology
ASC	Atypical squamous cells
ASCP	American Society for Clinical Pathology
ASCUS	Atypical squamous cells of undetermined significance
ASD	Atrial septal defect
ASR	Analyte specific reagent
CA	Cancer
CABG	Coronary artery bypass graft
CAP	College of American Pathologists
CDC	Centers for Disease Control and Prevention
CIN	Cervical intraepithelial neoplasia
CJD	Creutzfeldt-Jakob disease
CLIA '88	Clinical Laboratory Improvement Amendments of 1988
CMS	Centers for Medicare and Medicaid Services
CPC	Clinicopathologic conference
CQI	Continuous quality improvement
DCIS	Ductal carcinoma in situ
DRG	Diagnosis related groups
EM	Electron microscopy
EMS	Emergency medical services
ER	Estrogen receptor
FAD	Final autopsy diagnosis
FDA	US Food and Drug Administration
FISH	Fluorescence in situ hybridization

FMEA	Failure mode effects analysis
FN	False-negative
FNA	Fine-needle aspiration
FP	False-positive
FS	Frozen section
H&E	Hematoxylin and eosin
HHS	United States Department of Health and Human Services
HIPAA	Health Insurance Portability and Accountability Act of 1996
HIV	Human immunodeficiency virus
HPS	Hantavirus pulmonary syndrome
HPV	Human papillomavirus
HSIL	High-grade squamous intraepithelial lesion
ICD	International classification of diseases
IF	Immunofluorescence
IHC	Immunohistochemistry
IRB	Institutional review board
ISH	In situ hybridization
IVD	In vitro diagnostic use
JCAHO	Joint Commission on Accreditation of Healthcare Organizations
LAP	Laboratory Accreditation Program of the CAP
LOS	Length of stay
LSIL	Low-grade squamous intraepithelial lesion
M&M	Morbidity and mortality
MIME	Midwest Institute for Medical Education
NCCLS	Clinical and Laboratory Standards Institute (formerly NCCLS)
NEQAS	United Kingdom National External Quality Assessment Service
NOK	Next of kin
OSHA	Occupational Safety and Health Administration
PAD	Preliminary autopsy diagnosis
PIN	Prostatic intraepithelial neoplasia
QA	Quality assurance
QC	Quality control

QI	Quality improvement
QM	Quality management
RPN	Risk priority number
RUO	Research use only
SARS	Severe acute respiratory syndrome
SIDS	Sudden infant death syndrome
SIL	Squamous intraepithelial lesion
SNOMED	Systematized Nomenclature of Medicine
TAT	Turnaround time
TN	True-negative
TP	True-positive
TURP	Transurethral resection of the prostate
VA	Veterans Administration
VSD	Ventricular septal defect
WHO	World Health Organization